INTERVENTIONAL CARDIOLOGY CLINICS

www.interventional.theclinics.com

Consulting Editor

MARVIN H. ENG

Multi-Modality Interventional Imaging

January 2024 • Volume 13 • Number 1

Editor

Thomas W. Smith

ELSEVIER

1600 John F. Kennedy Boulevard • Suite 1800 • Philadelphia, Pennsylvania, 19103-2899

http://www.theclinics.com

INTERVENTIONAL CARDIOLOGY CLINICS Volume 13, Number 1
January 2024 ISSN 2211-7458, ISBN-13: 978-0-443-18352-2

Editor: Joanna Gascoine
Developmental Editor: Akshay Samson

Interventional Cardiology Clinics (ISSN 2211-7458) is published quarterly by Elsevier Inc., 360 Park Avenue South, New York, NY 10010-1710. Months of issue are January, April, July, and October. Subscription prices are USD 224 per year for US individuals, USD 100 per year for US students, USD 224 per year for Canadian individuals, USD 100 per year for Canadian students, USD 317 per year for international individuals, and USD 150 per year for international students. For institutional access pricing please contact Customer Service via the contact information below. To receive student/resident rate, orders must be accompanied by name of affiliated institution, date of term, and the *signature* of program/residency coordinator on institution letterhead. Orders will be billed at individual rate until proof of status is received. Foreign air speed delivery is included in all *Clinics* subscription prices. All prices are subject to change without notice. **POSTMASTER:** Send address changes to *Interventional Cardiology Clinics*, Elsevier Health Sciences Division, Subscription Customer Service, 3251 Riverport Lane, Maryland Heights, MO 63043. **Customer Service: Telephone: 1-800-654-2452** (U.S. and Canada); **1-314-447-8871** (outside U.S. and Canada). **Fax: 1-314-447-8029.** E-mail: journalscustomerservice-usa@elsevier.com (for print support); journalsonlinesupport-usa@elsevier.com (for online support).

Reprints. For copies of 100 or more of articles in this publication, please contact the Commercial Reprints Department, Elsevier Inc., 360 Park Avenue South, New York, NY 10010-1710. Tel.: 212-633-3874; Fax: 212-633-3820; E-mail: reprints@elsevier.com.

CONTRIBUTORS

CONSULTING EDITOR

MARVIN H. ENG, MD
Structural Heart Program Medical Director,
Structural Heart Disease Fellowship Director,
Director of Cardiovascular Quality, Banner
University Medical Center, Phoenix,
Arizona, USA

EDITOR

THOMAS W. SMITH, MD
Chief of Cardiology, Division of
Cardiovascular Medicine, Department of
Internal Medicine, University of California,
Davis Medical Center, Sacramento, California,
USA

AUTHORS

VRATIKA AGARWAL, MD
Division of Cardiology, Department of
Medicine, Columbia University Irving Medical
Center, NewYork-Presbyterian Hospital, New
York, New York, USA

EDRIS AMAN, MD
Associate Clinical Professor of Cardiovascular
Medicine, University of California, Davis
Medical Center, Sacramento, California,
USA

KWAME B. ATSINA, MD
Assistant Clinical Professor of Cardiovascular
Medicine, University of California, Davis
Medical Center, Sacramento, California,
USA

SENTHIL S. BALASUBRAMANIAN, MD
Division of Cardiology, Montefiore Medical
Center, Albert Einstein College of Medicine,
Bronx, New York, USA; Division of Cardiology,
University of Chicago, Northshore University
Health System, Evanston, Illinois,
USA

EDWARD CHAU, MD
Cardiovascular Fellow, Division of
Cardiovascular Medicine, University of
California, Davis Medical Center, Sacramento,
California, USA

TAM DOAN, MD
Assistant Professor of Pediatrics, Division of
Pediatric Cardiology, Coronary Artery
Anomalies Program, The Lillie Frank
Abercrombie Section of Cardiology,
Texas Children's Hospital, Baylor
College of Medicine, Houston, Texas,
USA

ADITYA DESAI, MD
Resident physician Department of Internal
Medicine, University of California, Riverside
School of Medicine, Riverside, California, USA

DARSHI DESAI, MD
Resident physician Department of Internal
Medicine, University of California, Riverside
School of Medicine, Riverside, California, USA

CARTER W. ENGLISH, MD
Advanced Cardiovascular Imaging Fellow,
Division of Cardiovascular Medicine,
Department of Internal Medicine, University of
California, Davis Medical Center, Sacramento,
California, USA

MARIO J. GARCIA, MD
Chief, Cardiology, Co-Director Division of
Cardiology, Montefiore Medical Center,
Professor Albert Einstein College of Medicine,
Bronx, New York, USA

SAFWAN GAZNABI, MD
Resident Physician Division of Cardiology, Montefiore Medical Center, Albert Einstein College of Medicine, Bronx, New York, USA; Division of Cardiology, University of Chicago, Northshore University Health System, Evanston, Illinois, USA

BASHAER GHEYATH, MD
Multimodality Cardiovascular Imaging Fellow, Department of Imaging, Cedars-Sinai Medical Center, Los Angeles, California, USA

CARLOS A. GONGORA, MD
Division of Cardiology, Montefiore Medical Center, Albert Einstein College of Medicine, Bronx, New York, USA

REBECCA HAHN, MD
Professor Division of Cardiology, Department of Medicine, Columbia University Irving Medical Center, NewYork-Presbyterian Hospital, New York, New York, USA

EDWIN C. HO, MD
Co-Director of the Heart Valve/Structural Heart Center Division of Cardiology, Montefiore Medical Center, Albert Einstein College of Medicine, Bronx, New York, USA

DAE-HEE KIM, MD, PhD
Associate Professor of Medicine, Division of Cardiology, Asan Medical Center, College of Medicine, University of Ulsan, Seoul, Korea

TAKESHI KITAI, MD, PhD, FHFSA
Director of Cardiovascular Care Unit, Department of Cardiovascular Medicine, Kobe City Medical Center General Hospital, Kobe, Japan

AZEEM LATIB, MD
Section Head and Director of Interventional Cardiology; Director of Structural Heart Interventions Division of Cardiology, Montefiore Medical Center, Albert Einstein College of Medicine, Bronx, New York, USA

SYED LATIF, MD
Cardiologist, Heart and Vascular Institute, Sutter Medical Center, Sacramento, California, USA

DANIEL LORENZATTI, MD
Research fellow, Division of Cardiology, Montefiore Medical Center, Albert Einstein College of Medicine, Bronx, New York, USA

JEIRYM MIRANDA, MD
Advanced Cardiac Imaging Fellow Division of Cardiology, Montefiore Medical Center, Albert Einstein College of Medicine, Bronx, New York, USA; Division of Cardiology, Mount Sinai, Morningside, New York, USA

SILVANA MOLOSSI, MD, PhD
Associate Professor of Pediatrics, Division of Pediatric Cardiology, Coronary Artery Anomalies Program, The Lillie Frank Abercrombie Section of Cardiology, Texas Children's Hospital, Baylor College of Medicine, Houston, Texas, USA

PANKAJ MALHOTRA, MD
Advanced Cardiac Imaging Fellow, Department of Imaging, Mark Taper Imaging Center, Smidt Heart Institute, Cedars-Sinai Medical Center, Los Angeles, California, USA

RHONDA MIYASAKA, MD
Department of Cardiovascular Medicine, Heart and Vascular Institute, Cleveland Clinic, Cleveland, Ohio, USA

MITSUHIKO OTA, MD
Department of Cardiovascular Center, Toranomon Hospital, Tokyo, Japan

TAI H. PHAM, MD
Structural Heart Disease Fellow Division of Cardiovascular Medicine, University of California, Davis Medical Center, Sacramento, California, USA Sacramento, California, USA

PURVI PARWANI, MBBS, MPH, FACC
Associate Professor of Medicine, Multimodality Cardiovascular Imager, Division of Cardiology, Department of Medicine, Loma Linda University Health, Loma Linda, California, USA

PAMELA PIÑA, MD
Division of Cardiology, Montefiore Medical Center, Albert Einstein College of Medicine, Bronx, New York, USA; Division of Cardiology, CEDIMAT, Santo Domingo, Dominican Republic

JAY RAMCHAND, MD, PhD
Department of Cardiovascular Medicine,
Heart and Vascular Institute, Cleveland Clinic,
Cleveland, Ohio, USA

JASON H. ROGERS, MD
Professor, Division of Cardiovascular
Medicine, Department of Internal
Medicine, University of California, Davis
Medical Center, Sacramento, California, USA

SHAGUN SACHDEVA, MD
Assistant Professor of Pediatrics,
Division of Pediatric Cardiology, Coronary
Artery Anomalies Program, The Lillie
Frank Abercrombie Section of Cardiology,
Texas Children's Hospital, Baylor
College of Medicine, Houston, Texas, USA

ANDREA SCOTTI, MD
Structural Heart Intervention Fellow Division
of Cardiology, Montefiore Medical Center,
Albert Einstein College of Medicine, Bronx,
New York, USA

ALDO L. SCHENONE, MD
Division of Cardiology, Montefiore Medical
Center, Albert Einstein College of Medicine,
Bronx, New York, USA

GAGAN D. SINGH, MD, FACC, FSCAI
Professor, Division of Cardiovascular
Medicine, University of California, Davis
Medical Center, Sacramento, California,
USA

LEANDRO SLIPCZUK, MD, PhD, FACC
Section Head, Director of Interventional
Cardiology; Director of Structural Heart
Interventions Division of Cardiology,
Montefiore Medical Center, Assistant
professor Albert Einstein College of Medicine,
Bronx, New York, USA

THOMAS W. SMITH, MD
Chief of Cardiology, Division of Cardiovascular
Medicine, Department of Internal Medicine,
University of California, Davis Medical Center,
Sacramento, California, USA

JAY RAMCHAND, MD, PhD
Department of Cardiovascular Medicine,
Heart and Vascular Institute, Cleveland Clinic,
Cleveland, Ohio, USA

JASON H. ROGERS, MD
Professor, Division of Cardiovascular
Medicine, Department of Internal
Medicine, University of California, Davis
Medical Center, Sacramento, California, USA

SHAGUN SACHDEVA, MD
Assistant Professor of Pediatrics,
Division of Pediatric Cardiology, Coronary
Artery Anomalies Program, The Lillie
Frank Abercrombie Section of Cardiology,
Texas Children's Hospital, Baylor
College of Medicine, Houston, Texas, USA

ANDREA SCOTTI, MD
Structural Heart Intervention Fellow, Division
of Cardiology, Montefiore Medical Center,
Albert Einstein College of Medicine, Bronx,
New York, USA

ALDO L. SCHENONE, MD
Division of Cardiology, Montefiore Medical
Center, Albert Einstein College of Medicine,
Bronx, New York, USA

GAGAN D. SINGH, MD, FACC, FSCAI
Professor, Division of Cardiovascular
Medicine, University of California, Davis
Medical Center, Sacramento, California,
USA

LEANDRO SLIPCZUK, MD, PhD, FACC
Section Head, Director of Interventional
Cardiology, Director of Structural Heart
Interventions Division of Cardiology,
Montefiore Medical Center, Assistant
professor Albert Einstein College of Medicine,
Bronx, New York, USA

THOMAS W. SMITH, MD
Chief of Cardiology, Division of Cardiovascular
Medicine, Department of Internal Medicine,
University of California, Davis Medical Center,
Sacramento, California, USA

CONTENTS

As transcatheter tricuspid interventions have emerged, especially edge-to-edge repair, imaging has shown to be key in optimizing transcatheter outcomes. Given the location of the tricuspid valve relative to the esophagus, transesophageal echocardiography has proven difficult and utilization of three-dimensional (3D) multiplanar reconstruction has become essential. Three-dimensional intracardiac echocardiography is a useful imaging adjunct for tricuspid edge-to-edge repair. As 3D intracardiac echocardiography evolves, it may supplant transesophageal echocardiography as the imaging modality of choice in transcatheter tricuspid valve interventions.

Transcatheter structural heart interventions are expanding into more complex spaces including mitral transcatheter edge-to-edge repair, left atrial appendage occlusion, tricuspid transcatheter edge-to-edge repair, mitral/tricuspid valve-in-valve, and perivalvular leak closures. Transesophageal echocardiography (TEE), with concomitant fluoroscopy, has remained the gold standard for many of these interventions. Although three-dimensional intracardiac echocardiography has been used, applications were often limited to guidance for more "simple" procedures such as patent foramen ovale/atrial septal defect closure and/or intraprocedural adjunctive imaging guidance. However, patients with an excessive risk for general anesthesia or contraindications to TEE, including esophageal/gastric disease, cervical/thoracic spinal disease, or coagulopathies, have limited options.

Transcatheter left atrial appendage occlusion (LAAO) is an alternative to systemic anticoagulation in patients with non-valvular atrial fibrillation with increased risk for thromboembolic events. Pre- and post-procedural imaging is essential for technical success, allowing practitioners to identify contraindications, select appropriate devices, and recognize procedural complications. Although transesophageal echocardiography has traditionally served as the preeminent imaging modality in LAAO, cardiac computed tomography imaging has emerged as a noninvasive surrogate given its excellent isotropic spatial resolution, multiplanar reconstruction capability, rapid temporal resolution, and large field of view.

With the increase in structural heart procedural volume, interventional imagers are required. Multiple imaging modalities exist to guide these procedures. With comprehensive understanding of pathology, anatomy, and procedures, an advanced imager plays an important role in the heart team. Imaging training is part of general cardiology fellowship. Current structures do not provide adequate procedural time to fill the role. Interested graduates pursue advanced training by either focusing on echocardiography and procedural imaging or multidetector computed tomography and cardiac magnetic resonance. This yields individuals with different expertise.

 Video content accompanies this article at http://www.interventional.theclinics.com.

Over the past decade, engineering advances in intracardiac echocardiography (ICE) have improved the ability of an imager or interventionalist to guide not only interatrial septal procedures but now commonly left atrial appendage, tricuspid, and mitral procedures. When transesophageal echocardiography (TEE) is not possible because of anatomic limitations, ICE has proved a useful tool to safely complete structural interventions. ICE will play a growing, key role in structural interventions where anatomic factors strongly favor an intracardiac perspective or augment TEE when imaging is suboptimal.

Congenital coronary anomalies are not an infrequent occurrence and their clinical presentation typically occurs during early years, though may be manifested only in adulthood. In the setting of anomalous aortic origin of a coronary artery, this is particularly concerning as it inflicts sudden loss of healthy young lives. Risk stratification remains a challenge and so does the best management decision-making in these patients, particularly if asymptomatic. Standardized approach to evaluation and management, with careful data collection and collaboration among centers, will likely impact future outcomes in this patient population, thus allowing for exercise participation and healthier lives.

Detailed preoperative and intraoperative echocardiographic assessment of the mitral valve apparatus is critical for a successful repair. The recent advent of 3-dimensional transesophageal echocardiography has added an extra pivotal role to transesophageal echocardiography in the assessment of mitral apparatus and mitral regurgitation. Because surgeons must rapidly decide whether cardiopulmonary bypass should be continued to be weaned off or a second pump run should be selected, the echocardiographer conducting intraoperative transesophageal echocardiography is required to be trained according to a certain algorithm. This review summarizes the current clinical role of intraoperative transesophageal echocardiography in mitral valve repair in the operating room.

During the last few years, there has been a substantial shift in efforts to understand and manage secondary or functional tricuspid regurgitation (TR) given its prevalence, adverse prognostic impact, and symptom burden associated with progressive right heart failure. Understanding the pathophysiology of TR and right heart failure is crucial for determining the best treatment strategy and improving outcomes. In this article, we review the complex relationship between right heart structural and hemodynamic changes that drive the pathophysiology of secondary TR and discuss the role of multimodality imaging in the diagnosis, management, and determination of outcomes.

Current guidelines of aortic stenosis (AS) management focus on valve parameters, LV systolic dysfunction, and symptoms; however, emerging data suggest that there may be benefit of aortic valve replacement before it becomes severe by present criteria. Myocardial assessment using novel multimodality imaging techniques exhibits subclinical myocardial injury and remodeling at various stages before guideline-directed interventions, which predicts adverse outcomes. This raises the question of whether implementing serial myocardial assessment should become part of the standard appraisal, thereby identifying high-risk patients aiming to minimize adverse outcomes.

Mitral valve disease is the most common valvular heart disease. Imaging determines the etiology (anatomic assessment), valve function and severity of valvular heart disease (hemodynamic assessment), remodeling of the left ventricle and right ventricle, and preplanning and guidance of percutaneous intervention. Although roles of computed tomography and magnetic resonance are increasing, echocardiography serves as the first-line imaging modality for the diagnosis and serial follow-up in most cases. This review summarizes the roles of multimodality imaging currently available from research fields to daily clinical practice.

Transcatheter edge-to-edge mitral valve repair is a minimally invasive treatment option for selected patients with moderate to severe or severe mitral regurgitation. Although transcatheter edge-to-edge mitral valve repair offers a significant step forward in the management of mitral regurgitation, the rate of procedural-related complications is not trivial. High-quality periprocedural imaging is important for optimal patient selection and procedural success. In this review, we present a step-by-step approach of the recommended echocardiographic views for transcatheter edge-to-edge mitral valve repair.

MULTI-MODALITY INTERVENTIONAL IMAGING

ISSUES OF RELATED INTEREST

Cardiology Clinics
https://www.cardiology.theclinics.com/
Cardiac Electrophysiology Clinics
http://www.cardiacep.theclinics.com/
Heart Failure Clinics
https://www.heartfailure.theclinics.com/

THE CLINICS ARE NOW AVAILABLE ONLINE!

Access your subscription at:
www.theclinics.com

FOREWORD

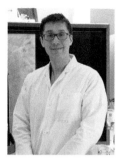

Marvin H. Eng, MD
Consulting Editor

We are pleased to introduce this issue of *Interventional Cardiology Clinics* that delves into the catalyst for the structural revolution, advanced cardiac imaging. The tools for characterizing cardiac anatomy have been present for some time, but the temporal and spatial resolution of 3D imaging has provided insights into cardiac structure that makes engineering and implanting devices more feasible than ever. Finally, application of multimodality imaging for device therapy has forged the growing niche of Interventional Imaging, now the cornerstone for structural interventions.

Advanced cardiac imaging has multiplied the role of characterization of the cardiac structure and function, especially for interventionalists. Engineering advances in sonographic probes and processor speeds have now brought real-time 3D imaging (4D) intracardiac. Intracardiac 4D imaging is the latest of tools interventionalists are learning to implement, and there is special weight to this advancement in our issue. Implementation of 4D imaging, both transesophageal and intracardiac echocardiography, is thoroughly explained by world-class interventional imagers. Furthermore, the training pathways and career development of advanced imaging are discussed by our guest editor.

Thomas Smith, a senior advanced imager and chief of cardiology, edited this issue of *Interventional Cardiology Clinics*. We congratulate Dr Smith for this illuminating issue that captures the recent progress in Interventional Cardiac Imaging.

Marvin H. Eng, MD
Banner University Medical Center
1111 East McDowell Road
Phoenix, AZ 85006, USA

E-mail address:
marvin.eng@bannerhealth.com

https://doi.org/10.1016/j.iccl.2023.10.001
2211-7458/24/© 2023 Published by Elsevier Inc.

Tricuspid Valve Transcatheter Edge-To-Edge Repair Guidance with Transesophageal Echocardiography and Intracardiac Echocardiography

Edris Aman, MD*, Kwame B. Atsina, MD

KEYWORDS

- Tricuspid regurgitation • Transcatheter tricuspid valve repair
- Transcatheter edge-to-edge repair (TEER) • Transesophageal echocardiography (TEE)
- Intracardiac echocardiography (ICE) • Multiplanar reconstruction (MPR)
- Interventional echocardiography

KEY POINTS

- Tricuspid valve anatomy is variable and complex, which increases the importance of adequate echocardiographic imaging to guide tricuspid transcatheter edge-to-edge repair (TEER).
- Transesophageal echocardiography (TEE) can be suboptimal in tricuspid imaging, given the relationship of esophagus to tricuspid valve.
- Multiplanar reconstruction is critical for TEE imaging to guide tricuspid edge-to-edge repair.
- Intracardiac echocardiography can assess for adequate leaflet insertion when TEE views are limited.

INTRODUCTION

Tricuspid regurgitation has been shown to be independently associated with increased mortality.[1] Nevertheless, isolated tricuspid surgery is infrequently performed because it is associated with high surgical mortality.[2,3] This need for intervention has spurred innovation leading to new transcatheter valve interventions.[4,5] Intraprocedural imaging is key to perform these new transcatheter tricuspid valve interventions safely and effectively.

This review will describe tricuspid valve anatomy, cause of tricuspid regurgitation, preprocedure transesophageal echocardiography (TEE), and key intraprocedural TEE views that guide tricuspid transcatheter edge-to-edge repair

(TEER). We will also describe the indications and use of intracardiac echocardiography (ICE) as an adjunct imaging modality during tricuspid TEER.

TRICUSPID VALVE ANATOMY

Tricuspid valve anatomy is variable and complex, and anatomic understanding is key to guiding interventional procedures via TEE or ICE.[6] The tricuspid valve apparatus contains leaflets, chordae tendinae, and papillary muscles. The tricuspid valve, as traditionally taught, has 3 leaflets: septal, anterior, and posterior. The anterior leaflet is the largest and most superiorly oriented leaflet. The posterior leaflet is usually the smallest in annular circumference and has

---

University of California, Davis Medical Center, 4860 Y Street, Suite 0200, Sacramento, CA 95817, USA
* Corresponding author.
E-mail address: eaman@ucdavis.edu

Intervent Cardiol Clin 13 (2024) 1–10
https://doi.org/10.1016/j.iccl.2023.08.004
2211-7458/24/

multiple scallops.[7] More recent literature has revealed that there are often more than 3 leaflets, and a naming nomenclature to account for the multiple leaflets ($\geq$4) has been proposed.[8] There are at least 2 papillary muscles (anterior and posterior) and a variable third papillary muscle (septal). The anterior papillary muscle provides chordae to the anterior and posterior leaflets and originates from the anterolateral wall of the right ventricle. The anterior papillary muscle distinguishes the anterior and posterior leaflets. The posterior papillary muscle provides chordae to the posterior and septal leaflets.[9]

Structural abnormalities in the tricuspid valve apparatus can lead to incomplete coaptation of the tricuspid leaflets and resultant tricuspid regurgitation. In addition to abnormalities in the tricuspid apparatus, enlargement of the right atrium or right ventricle can cause tricuspid annular dilatation with resultant tricuspid regurgitation.[10]

TRICUSPID REGURGITATION ETIOLOGY

Cause of tricuspid regurgitation is broadly categorized into primary, secondary, and cardiac implantable electronic device (CIED)-induced tricuspid regurgitation.

Primary tricuspid regurgitation, accounting for 10% to 15% of patients, is due to leaflet pathologic condition: prolapse, flail, Ebstein anomaly, leaflet clefts, rheumatic disease, infective endocarditis, carcinoid disease, and so forth.

Secondary tricuspid regurgitation, accounting for ~80% of patients, involves normal leaflet morphology with regurgitation occurring from annular dilatation and/or leaflet tethering. Secondary tricuspid regurgitation can be due to atrial or ventricular dilatation. Atrial secondary tricuspid regurgitation is a diagnosis of exclusion, absence of leaflet abnormality, LV dysfunction, left-sided valve disease, pulmonary hypertension, or CIED.[11] Patients with atrial-induced tricuspid regurgitation typically have a long-standing atrial fibrillation with marked right atrial enlargement.[12] In this setting, the tricuspid annulus becomes more planar and is larger than cases of primary or ventricular secondary tricuspid regurgitation.[13] Ventricular secondary tricuspid regurgitation is due to primary pulmonary hypertension or secondary pulmonary hypertension (left heart disease, chronic lung disease, pulmonary thromboembolism, and left-to-right shunt) resulting in ventricular dilatation. The ventricular dilatation leads to leaflet tethering, restricted motion in systole, and possibly right atrial dilatation.[14]

CIED-induced tricuspid regurgitation accounts for ~5% of patients. Primary CIED-induced tricuspid regurgitation is caused by direct interaction of CIED leads with valve leaflets.[15,16]

Understanding the cause of tricuspid regurgitation is a key goal of preprocedure TEE.

PREPROCEDURE TRANSESOPHAGEAL ECHOCARDIOGRAPHY

The tricuspid valve is anterior, and thus, it is further from the esophagus than the mitral or aortic valve. Given the location of the tricuspid valve, multiple acoustic windows must be used for optimal imaging. The goal of preprocedure TEE is to determine the cause of tricuspid regurgitation.

Zero-degree Omniplane

We begin preprocedure TEE at a 0° omniplane and advance the probe in to move from the anterior to posterior aspect of the tricuspid valve (Fig. 1). We evaluate the tricuspid valve with two-dimensional (2D) imaging and color Doppler, ensuring the Nyquist limit is at least 50 cm/s. The 2D 0° evaluation is key for mid and deep esophageal imaging because it allows the imager to determine the best level to image the tricuspid valve. Oftentimes, the deep esophageal view provides the highest image quality. Once identified, the omniplane can be changed while maintaining the optimal level of depth.

Tricuspid "Bicom" View

When an acoustic window is found at 0°, which provides an optimal view of the tricuspid valve, the omniplane can be increased to 60° to 80° to create the right ventricular (RV) inflow view or "bicom" view of the valve (Fig. 2). This view dissects the tricuspid valve parallel to the line of coaptation between the anterior and posterior leaflets and the septal leaflet. To ensure the plane is truly parallel to the desired line of coaptation, the use of live 3D imaging can confirm the imaging plane. Once the "bicom" view is confirmed, biplane imaging can be used to view the septal-anterior leaflets when the tilt plane is moved closer to the aortic valve and to view the septal-posterior leaflets when the tilt plane is moved away from the aortic valve (Fig. 3). The transition from septal-anterior to septal-posterior can be difficult to view because the tricuspid valve is often composed of more than 3 leaflets. Thus, the transgastric view is essential to evaluate tricuspid valve leaflet morphology.

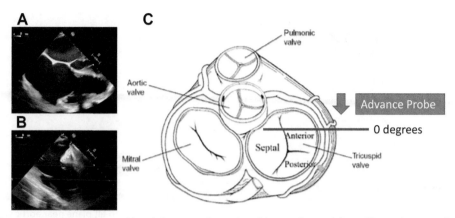

Fig. 1. Images *A* and *B* are from mid and deep esophageal positions at 0° omniplane. The probe was advanced in to move from images A to B and retracted to move images B to A. Image *C* is an anatomic figure of the heart. Zero-degree omniplane dissects the tricuspid valve at septal-anterior leaflets at mid-esophageal position and septal-posterior leaflets at the deep esophageal position. Advancing the TEE probe allows you to evaluate move from the anterior to posterior part of the tricuspid valve.

Transgastric

The transgastric view is essential to understand tricuspid valve leaflets. It is the only 2D view that provides visualization of all leaflets at the same time. In order to obtain the transgastric view, the probe should be advanced into a gastric position and anteflexed. The omniplane should then be increased to 20° to 60°. Subtle clockwise rotation of the probe can then be applied to ensure leaflet tip coaptation is being viewed (Fig. 4). With this view, the number of leaflets, clefts, and coaptation gaps can be accurately measured.

Three-dimensional Imaging

From any 2D acoustic window, 3D datasets can be obtained. The quality of 3D datasets depends on the quality of 2D images. Thus, 3D datasets should be obtained from the best 2D acoustic window. Initial 3D imaging can be focused on the tricuspid valve (Fig. 5). Multiplanar reconstruction (MPR) should be done if the initial 3D imaging is of good quality. MPR allows the imager to generate the RV inflow, 4 chamber, and short axis views of the tricuspid valve. Rotation of the plane in the short axis view can allow the imager to see the true grasp view for edge-to-edge repair (Fig. 6). Coaptation gaps can be evaluated in the short axis view as well. This influences the decision on what type on transcatheter intervention to perform (repair vs replacement).[17]

PROCEDURAL IMAGE GUIDANCE WITH TRANSESOPHAGEAL ECHOCARDIOGRAPHY

Introduction of Steerable Guide Catheter into Right Atrium

A guidewire is placed from the inferior vena cava (IVC) into the superior vena cava (SVC). The

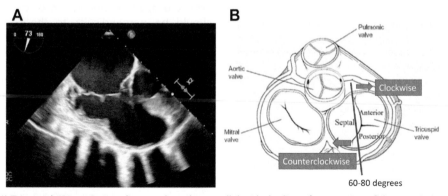

Fig. 2. (*A*) Tricuspid "Bicom" view dissects the valve parallel with the line of coaptation of the anterior and posterior leaflets with the septal leaflet. (*B*) Anatomic figure demonstrating how omniplane slices the tricuspid valve. Clockwise rotation of probe moves acoustic window laterally and counter-clockwise rotation of probe moves acoustic window septally.

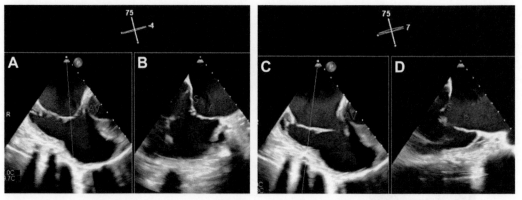

Fig. 3. Biplane imaging. (A) RV inflow-outflow view obtained at 75° omniplane with tilt plane near aortic valve (AV). (B) X-plane view demonstrating the septal and anterior leaflets. (C) RV inflow-outflow view obtained at 75° omniplane with tilt plane far away from AV. (D) X-plane view demonstrating the septal and posterior leaflets.

steerable guide catheter (SGC) is then advanced over the guidewire. The guidewire is then removed. At this time, the SGC is oriented away from the interatrial septum and retracted to the lower third of the right atrium. The imaging for this portion of the procedure is done primarily in a bicaval view or in a bicaval view with biplane imaging (Fig. 7).

Clip Delivery System

The clip delivery system (CDS) is then advanced through the SGC. Initial imaging is done in a bicaval view, and the omniplane is adjusted in order to focus on the tip of the CDS. Careful imaging is key to avoid injury to the interatrial septum as the CDS is guided antero-inferiorly toward the tricuspid valve. As the CDS moves anteriorly, the probe should be rotated counter-clockwise and the omniplane adjusted

to focus on the CDS. As the CDS move inferiorly toward the tricuspid valve, biplane imaging should be used to simultaneously visualize the anterior-posterior trajectory via RV inflow view, and septal-lateral trajectory via 4-chamber view (Fig. 8). This use of biplane allows the interventionalist to move the CDS and understand its location in 3D space.

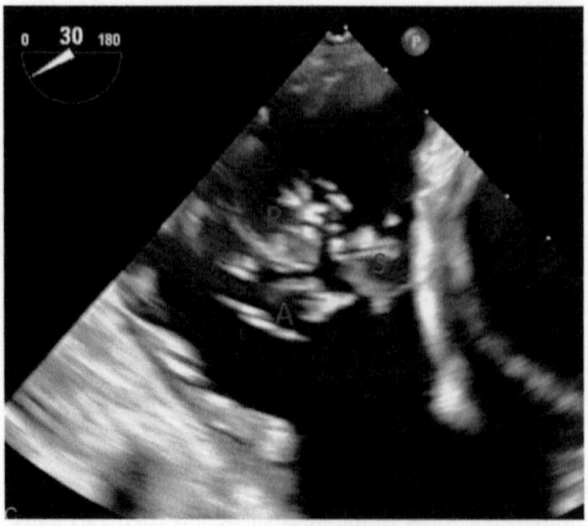

If conventional 2D TEE imaging is suboptimal, the imager can use one good acoustic window to create an RV inflow and 4-chamber view with 3D MPR. Using 3D MPR, the imager can still continue to provide procedural image guidance with minimal probe manipulation. This can be a good option for patients with known esophageal varices or predisposition to bleeding.

Clip Delivery System Trajectory and Clip Alignment Above Tricuspid Valve

The CDS trajectory is assessed with biplane imaging from the RV inflow view (see Fig. 8). Once trajectory is deemed acceptable, the clip arms are opened. Orientation of the clip arms should be perpendicular to the segment of coaptation gap. This can be assessed via 3 views: transgastric, 3D en-face, or 3D MPR. We will often assess alignment via 3D MPR as it allows for real-time evaluation of the CDS trajectory, alignment, advancement into the RV, and leaflet grasp with minimal probe manipulation (Fig. 9), thus lowering the risk of TEE-related esophageal injury.[18]

Advancing Clip Delivery System into Right Ventricle

The CDS can be advanced into the right ventricle using biplane imaging from the RV inflow view or 3D MPR (Fig. 10). Advancement of CDS should be done carefully to avoid injury to the tricuspid

Fig. 4. Transgastric view demonstrating a trileaflet tricuspid valve. S, septal; A, anterior; and P, posterior.

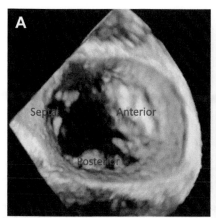 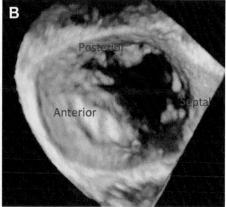

Fig. 5. (A) A 3D focused view of the tricuspid valve revealing trileaflet tricuspid valve in anatomic orientation. (B) A 3D focused view of the tricuspid valve oriented similar to transgastric view.

valve apparatus, specifically chordae and papillary muscle. Once in position, the clip arms are reopened and again the alignment is confirmed. Alignment confirmation beneath the valve is done using 3D en-face with lowering gain, 3D MPR, or transgastric views.

Grasping the Leaflets and Verification of Adequate Leaflet Insertion

Once alignment is confirmed, the clip arms of the CDS are lifted toward the tricuspid leaflets.

Leaflet grasping and verification of adequate leaflet insertion are integral to optimal patient outcomes.

Dedicated transgastric imaging can be performed in which the clip arms are fully imaged and leaflet motion is also captured. The sector width should be narrowed, and a long loop length recorded for postgrasp leaflet assessment. Focus should be paid to the leaflet just adjacent to the clip arms. As the grippers of the CDS are lowered, the leaflets within the

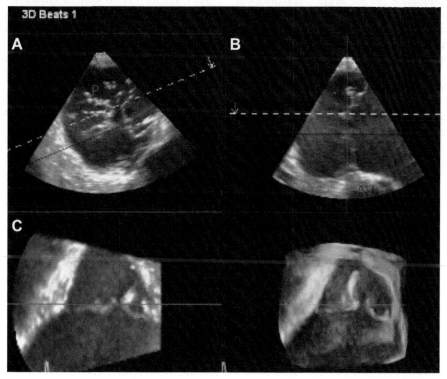

Fig. 6. (A) Short axis view of the tricuspid valve. (B) RV inflow-outflow view. (C) Grasp view, ideal for edge-to-edge repair, revealing septal and anterior leaflets. S, septal; A, anterior; P, posterior; AV, aortic valve.

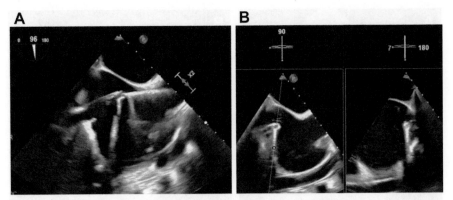

Fig. 7. (A) Bicaval view demonstrates SGC catheter, being positioned in the right atrium, with guidewire extending into the SVC. (B) Bicaval with biplane imaging to ensure SGC catheter is in optimal position before CDS introduction.

clip arms will become taut and seem to dive into the middle of the clip. Grasping can be confirmed through the review of the long loop acquisition, assessment of leaflet length in 3D MPR, or, if imaging permits, assessment of leaflet length in the biplane RV inflow view (Fig. 11). Before intervention, we will often measure the leaflet length at the site of potential clipping. Comparison of the leaflet length after intervention to the baseline is key to ensuring that an adequate leaflet length was grasped. Three-dimensional imaging is used to ensure an adequate orientation of the clips arms to the coaptation zone. Moreover, color Doppler assessment can also ensure there is no diastolic flow at the clip arms. These different assessments, long loop review, leaflet length preintervention and postintervention, 3D imaging to assess clip orientation, and color Doppler, are wholly used to ensure that an adequate length

of the leaflet has been grasped before deployment. Furthermore, a tricuspid inflow gradient is assessed before clip deployment. Given the large size of the tricuspid valve at baseline, gradients rarely exceed 5 mm Hg. 3D MPR can also be used to measure tricuspid valve area and 3D vena contacta area (VCA); it is an excellent technique for assessing edge-to-edge repair success after intervention.

Following clip release, we use biplane imaging from the RV inflow view to ensure the CDS is safely retracted into the SGC. The tricuspid valve is again assessed after clip deployment to ensure clip stability. Residual tricuspid regurgitation is assessed, and the strategy for subsequent clips is assessed. Residual tricuspid regurgitation, in our experience, is best evaluated with 3D VCA. A 3D MPR or transgastric imaging is key to determine if and where subsequent clips should be placed.

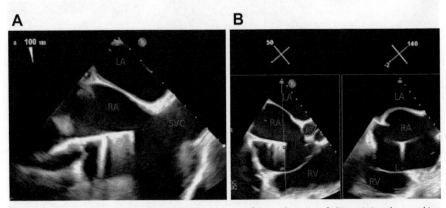

Fig. 8. Advancing CDS toward tricuspid valve. (A) Bicaval view focused on tip of clip as it is advanced into the right atrium. (B) Bicaval view with biplane imaging focused on tip of clip. LA, left atrium; RA, right atrium; SVC, superior vena cava; AV, aortic valve; RV, right ventricle; S, septal; L, lateral.

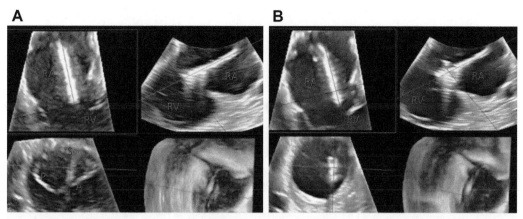

A   **B**

Fig. 9. (A) A 3D MPR demonstrating adequate trajectory before advancing into right ventricle. (B) A 3D MPR demonstrating proper clip alignment. The blue plane seen in RV inflow and grasp view can be lowered to leaflet to ensure clip is perpendicular to coaptation line. RA, right atrium; RV, right ventricle; S, septal; A, anterior; P, posterior.

INTRACARDIAC ECHOCARDIOGRAPHY

Given the difficulty in TEE imaging for triscuspid valve TEER, 3D ICE has emerged as an adjunct modality during cases.[19] There are currently 3 different 3D ICE catheters on the market.[20–22] We will not discuss the strengths and limitations of each ICE catheter in this article. Instead, we will discuss the basic use of 3D ICE in tricuspid TEER.

In order to use 3D ICE to its full capability, an understanding of biplane imaging and MPR is essential. When using 3D ICE, often the imager will need to recreate images ideally obtained in TEE. Because the ICE catheter emerges from the IVC and is manipulated antero-inferiorly to the tricuspid valve, an RV inflow view is initially obtained. The use of X-plane from this view creates a potential grasp view. A 3D volume can

then be obtained, and a 3D MPR can be used (Fig. 12).

Three-dimensional ICE can also be used for trajectory and alignment similar to TEE (Fig. 13). The greatest utility of 3D ICE is with leaflet insertion in edge-to-edge repair (Fig. 14). The limitation of TEE imaging, due to shadowing from mitral/aortic prosthesis, septal hypertrophy, and so forth, is especially problematic when assessing for leaflet insertion. Thus, 3D ICE, in our experience, has had the greatest utility in assessing leaflet insertion.

The strengths and limitations of TEE and 3D ICE are listed in Table 1. Understanding the strengths and limitations of TEE and 3D ICE is essential for determining when 3D ICE should be used, especially given the cost of these single-use catheters. At this time, 3D ICE does not have the technological capability to supplant TEE but as 3D ICE technology evolves, it may become the imaging modality of choice in tricuspid valve interventions.

DISCUSSION

Tricuspid valve imaging is difficult due to many factors. TEE imaging has improved with evolving technologies, the use of 3D imaging and in particular MPR. Using MPR, tricuspid TEER can be done from one acoustic window if 2D imaging is optimal enough. Understanding MPR is essential for the imager involved in a tricuspid TEER case. When TEE is suboptimal, 3D ICE can be used for trajectory, alignment, and even leaflet grasping. Three-dimensional ICE technology will need to evolve further but as it does, it may supplant TEE for tricuspid valve interventions.

Fig. 10. RV inflow with biplane imaging demonstrates clip arms opening below the tricuspid valve following advancement of CDS system into the right ventricle.

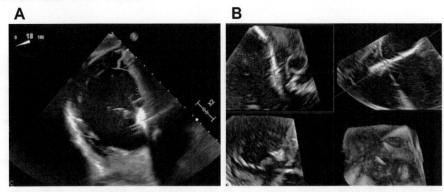

Fig. 11. (A) Transgastric imaging demonstrates taut septal and anterior leaflets diving into the clip. (B) A 3D MPR demonstrating clip at commissural septal-anterior position. S, septal; A, anterior.

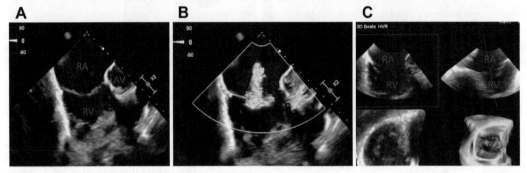

Fig. 12. A 3D intracardiac echocardiography. (A) RV inflow-outflow view obtained at 0°. (B) RV inflow-outflow view with color Doppler. (C) A 3D MPR. RA, right atrium; RV, right ventricle; S, septal; A, anterior; P, posterior.

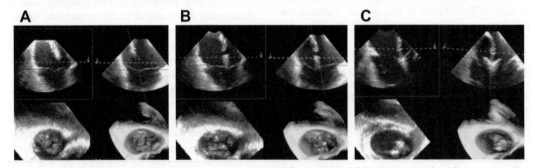

Fig. 13. Assessing trajectory and alignment using 3D MPR from 3D/4D ICE. (A) An initial evaluation revealing anterior trajectory of CDS. (B) Trajectory not corrected and CDS appears to be at central aspect of tricuspid valve. (C) Clip arms opened and alignment of arms relative to leaflets assessed.

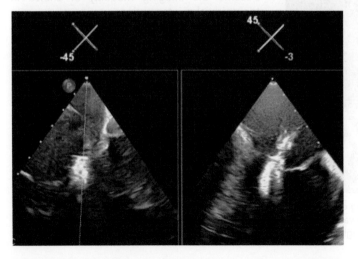

Fig. 14. Assessing leaflet insertion. (A) If an RV inflow/outflow (tricuspid "bicom") view is obtained with the clip directly under the transducer beam, then biplane imaging can provide a grasp view to assess for leaflet insertion.

Table 1
Strengths and limitations of TEE and 3D ICE for tricuspid TEER

	Transesophageal Echocardiography	Intracardiac Echocardiography
Strengths	• Superior visualization of far field structures • No change in temporal resolution with color Doppler • Orthogonal and 3D field of view 90 × 90° • TEE probe reusable and thus lower cost compared with 3D ICE	• Closer to tricuspid valve • If 3D ICE is only imaging modality in use, then can avoid general anesthesia • The avoidance of general anesthesia may contribute to faster postprocedure recovery, shorter hospital stay and lower costs overall
Limitations	• Risk of gatrointestinal trauma • Need for general anesthesia • Anatomic challenge of esophageal imaging due to distance from tricuspid valve	• Limited MPR orthogonal and 3D field of view • High cost of single-use catheters • Bleeding risk due to venous access

CLINICS CARE POINTS

- Careful screening TEE imaging is key to allow proper pre-intervention planning
- Utilization of 3D MPR, and possibly 3D ICE, is important as tricuspid valve acoustic windows can be limited

DECLARATION OF INTERESTS

Dr E. Aman has served as a consultant or received honoraria from Philips Healthcare, Siemens, and Abbott Structural. Dr K.B.Atsina has served as a consultant for Abbott Structural and MedTecX.

ACKNOWLEDGMENTS

The authors would like to acknowledge the contributions of Dr Thomas WR Smith, Dr Jason H. Rogers, and Dr Gagan Singh in developing our tricuspid valve intervention program.

REFERENCES

1. Chorin E, Rozenbaum Z, Topilsky Y, et al. Tricuspid regurgitation and long-term clinical outcomes. Eur Heart J Cardiovasc Imaging 2020;21:157–65.
2. Enriquez-Sarano M, Messika-Zeitoun D, Topilsky Y, et al. Tricuspid regurgitation is a public health crisis. Prog Cardiovasc Dis 2019;62:447–51.
3. Zack CJ, Fender EA, Chandrashekar P, et al. National trends and outcomes in isolated tricuspid valve surgery. J Am Coll Cardiol 2017;70:2953–60.
4. Lurz P, Stephan von Bardeleben R, Weber M, et al. TRILUMINATE Investigators. Transcatheter Edge-to-Edge Repair for Treatment of Tricuspid Regurgitation. J Am Coll Cardiol 2021;77(3):229–39.
5. Baldus S, Schofer N, Hausleiter J, et al. Transcatheter valve repair of tricuspid regurgitation with the PASCAL system: TriCLASP study 30-day results. Catheter Cardiovasc Interv 2022;100:1291–9.
6. Shah PM, Raney AA. Tricuspid valve disease. Curr Probl Cardiol 2008;33:47–84.
7. Ancona F, Agricola E, Stella S, et al. Interventional imaging of the tricuspid valve. Interv Cardiol Clin 2018;7:13–29.
8. Hahn Rebecca T, Weckbach Ludwig T, Noack Thilo, et al. Proposal for a Standard Echocardiographic Tricuspid Valve Nomenclature. JACC (J Am Coll Cardiol): Cardiovascular Imaging 2021;14:1299–305.
9. Aktas EO, Govsa F, Kocak A, et al. Variations in the papillary muscles of normal tricuspid valve and their clinical relevance in medicolegal autopsies. Saudi Med J 2004;25:1176–85.
10. Huttin O, Voilliot D, Mandry D, et al. All you need to know about the tricuspid valve: tricuspid valve imaging and tricuspid regurgitation analysis. Arch Cardiovasc Dis 2016;109:67–80.
11. Otto CM, Nishimura RA, Bonow RO, et al. ACC/AHA guideline for the management of patients with valvular heart disease: executive summary: a report of the American College of Cardiology/American Heart Association Joint Committee on Clinical Practice Guidelines. J Am Coll Cardiol 2021;77:450–500.
12. Muraru D, Addetia K, Guta AC, et al. Right atrial volume is a major determinant of tricuspid annulus area in functional tricuspid regurgitation: a three-dimensional echocardiographic study. Eur Heart J Cardiovasc Imaging 2021;22:660–9.
13. Muraru D, Caravita S, Guta AC, et al. Functional tricuspid regurgitation and atrial fibrillation: which comes first, the chicken or the egg? CASE 2020;4:458–63.

14. Hahn Rebecca T, Badano Luigi P, Bartko Philipp E, et al. recent advances in understanding pathophysiology, severity grading and outcome. European Heart Journal - Cardiovascular Imaging 2022;23(7):913–29.

15. Addetia K, Harb SC, Hahn RT, et al. Cardiac implantable electronic device lead-induced tricuspid regurgitation. JACC Cardiovasc Imaging 2019;12:622–36.

16. Polewczyk A, Kutarski A, Tomaszewski A, et al. Lead dependent tricuspid dysfunction: analysis of the mechanism and management in patients referred for transvenous lead extraction. Cardiol J 2013;20:402–10.

17. Ruf TF, Hahn RT, Kreidel F, et al. Short term clinical outcomes of transcatheter tricuspid valve repair with the third generation MitraClip XTR system. JACC Cardiovasc Interv 2021;14:1231–40.

18. Freitas-Ferraz Afonso B, Bernier Mathieu, Vaillancourt Rosaire, et al. Frédéric Nicodème, Jean-Michel Paradis, Jean Champagne, Gilles O'Hara, Lucia Junquera, David del Val, Guillem Muntané-Carol, Kim O'Connor, Jonathan Beaudoin, Josep Rodés-Cabau. Safety of Transesophageal Echocardiography to Guide Structural Cardiac Interventions. J Am Coll Cardiol 2020;75(25):3164–73.

19. Chadderdon S, Eleid MF, Thaden JM, et al. Three-Dimensional Intracardiac Echocardiography for Tricuspid Transcatheter Edge-to-Edge Repair. Structural Heart 2022;6(4).

20. Kaplan RM, Narang A, Gay H, et al. Use of a novel 4D intracardiac echocardiography catheter to guide interventional electrophysiology procedures. J Cardiovasc Electrophysiol 2021;32(12):3117–24.

21. Flautt Thomas, Da-Wariboko Akanibo, Lador Adi, et al. Left atrial appendage occlusion without fluoroscopy: optimization by 4d intracardiac echocardiography. JACC Cardiovasc Interv 2022;15(15):1592–4.

22. Ranard LS, Khalique OK, Donald E, et al. Transcatheter left atrial appendage closure using preprocedural computed tomography and intraprocedural 4-dimensional intracardiac echocardiography. Circ Cardiovasc Interv 2021;14(7):e010686.

3D Intracardiac Echocardiography for Structural Heart Interventions

Tai H. Pham, MD, Gagan D. Singh, MD*

KEYWORDS
• Intracardiac echocardiography • Structural heart • Transesophageal echocardiography

KEY POINTS
• Although considered the gold standard for imaging guidance for many structural heart procedures, numerous relative and absolute contraindications limit the utilization of transesophageal echocardiography (TEE).
• Three-dimensional (3D) intracardiac echocardiography (ICE) has been shown to be a safe and feasible option to guide structural heart interventions such as mitral-transcatheter edge-to-edge repair, left atrial appendage occlusion, perivalvular leak closure, and other complex structural interventions that require high fidelity real-time imaging guidance.
• Consideration of 3D ICE-guided structural heart interventions and its role when TEE remains an option is unclear and under investigation.

INTRODUCTION

Catheter-based ultrasound imaging technology has been explored for some time but it was not until the early 2000s that it was adopted for imaging guidance for structural heart interventions, predominantly with patent foramen ovale (PFO) and atrial septal defect (ASD) closures due to the excellent imaging windows of the interatrial septum.[1] Transcatheter structural heart interventions have evolved rapidly since then and continue to expand into more complex spaces including mitral transcatheter edge-to-edge repair (M-TEER), left atrial appendage occlusion (LAAO), tricuspid TEER, mitral/tricuspid valve-in-valve, and perivalvular leak (PVL) closures, to name a few. Transesophageal echocardiography (TEE), with concomitant fluoroscopy, has remained the gold standard for many of these interventions.[2] Although three-dimensional intracardiac echocardiography (3D ICE) has been used, applications were often limited to guidance for more "simple" procedures such as

PFO/ASD closure and/or intraprocedural adjunctive imaging guidance. However, in patients with an excessive risk for general anesthesia or contraindications to TEE, including esophageal/gastric disease, cervical/thoracic spinal disease, or coagulopathies, options have been limited. More recently, with the rapid improvement in quality of several platforms and ability to perform multiplanar reconstruction, 3D ICE has been used as an alternative with a high degree of procedural success. In this review, we evaluate the technical considerations and current data regarding 3D ICE-guidance within the evolving field of structural cardiology.

TECHNIQUE

There is no clear consensus or standardized imaging techniques with 3D ICE among current professional societies as there are with TEE. Earlier publications have well outlined the standard right-sided two-dimensional (2D) imaging windows (Fig. 1A and B) and the maneuvers

Division of Cardiovascular Medicine, University of California, Davis, 4860 Y Street, Suite 2820, Sacramento, CA 95817, USA
* Corresponding author.
E-mail address: drsingh@ucdavis.edu

Intervent Cardiol Clin 13 (2024) 11–17
https://doi.org/10.1016/j.iccl.2023.08.005

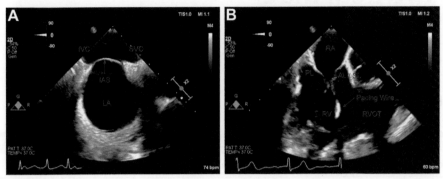

Fig. 1. RA views. (A) Mid-RA position with posterior flexion and gentle clockwise rotation reveals the "long-axis view" of the IAS. (B) With the probe in the lower RA at the neutral position, the "home view" allows for imaging of the TV, RV, and RVOT. AL, anterior leaflet; IAS, interatrial septum; IVC, inferior vena cava; LA, left atrium; PL, posterior leaflet; RA, right atrium; RV, right ventricle; RVOT, right ventricular outflow tract; SVC, superior vena cava.

required to achieve them.[3] With current generation 3D ICE catheters, it can be challenging to guide left-sided structural heart procedures with the catheter residing within the right atrium (RA). Hence, it is important to be able to successfully and safely navigate the 3D ICE catheter into the left atrium (LA) for intraprocedural guidance. This is achieved through direct placement of the catheter into the LA via a transseptal puncture with 1 of 2 techniques. A targeted transseptal puncture is performed under 3D ICE guidance. Next, the septal puncture is expanded to allow the advancement of the 3D ICE catheter into the LA under fluoroscopic guidance. This can be performed via several means: (1) dilatation with a standard 6–10 mm balloon or (2) advancement of the therapy catheter (eg, LAAO or TEER sheath) across the septum and back several times. Once the dilatation has occurred, using orthogonal fluoroscopic projections, the 3D ICE catheter is aligned with the preexisting LA rail wire, and it is advanced alongside the wire into the LA. The therapy system can then be advanced over the wire and into the LA. The second technique is with dual transseptal punctures. The challenge of performing 2 targeted transseptal punctures is often weighed against the benefits of creating a small ASD with less residual shunting. Experience with obtaining the above views and understanding the anatomy of various windows allow the operator to successfully guide many of the current structural heart interventions.

MITRAL TRANSCATHETER EDGE-TO-EDGE REPAIR

M-TEER is a viable option for patients with primary mitral regurgitation (MR) who are at a prohibitive risk for surgery.[4] Furthermore, in patients with moderate-to-severe MR who remain symptomatic despite maximally tolerated guideline-directed medical therapy, M-TEER has been shown to reduce heart failure hospitalizations and all-cause mortality.[5] Success of this procedure requires high-fidelity, real-time, intraprocedural imaging for optimal transseptal puncture guidance, device steering, and clip positioning. TEE with concomitant fluoroscopy has been the exclusive imaging modality for procedural guidance for the greater than 250,000 procedures performed worldwide and remains the gold standard.[2,6] In cases where TEE is prohibitive, 3D ICE is a reasonable alternative in highly select patients and anatomy.[7,8]

Procedural guidance with 3D ICE is similar to TEE short of a few differences. After advancement of the imaging catheter into the RA via femoral venous approach, targeted transseptal puncture is performed within the superior/mid aspect and posterior aspect of the fossa ovalis in the standard bicaval and short axis views. Transseptal puncture height is measured from the transseptal tent to the mitral annulus, often using an indirect sweep method because it can be difficult to get a tenting view and mitral valve (MV) in the same plane or using the multiplanar reconstruction feature on the console. After transseptal puncture, an LA rail wire is advanced into the LA. Balloon septostomy or catheter floss technique is performed to facilitate crossing of the 3D ICE catheter (as described above) and MitraClip steerable guide catheter (SGC) into the LA. From there, the assessment of MR severity, location, and mechanism can be confirmed from an earlier transthoracic echocardiography (TTE) with 2D, 3D, and multiplanar reconstruction. Spectral Doppler can be used to assess MV inflow gradient and pulmonary

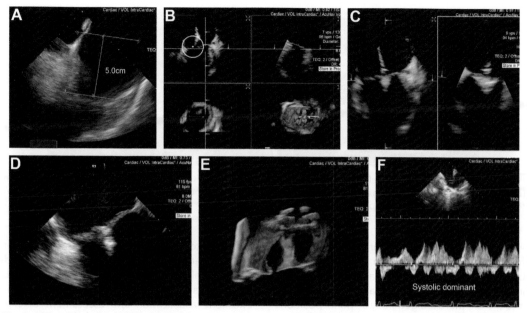

Fig. 2. ICE-guided mitral TEER. (A) Mid-RA view with sweep guiding for targeted transseptal puncture. (B) Direct LA view with MPR for supravalvular alignment and trajectory. (C) Direct LA view with X-plane for subvalvular alignment. Images (D and E) show deployed clip from the LA in the bicommissural view and 3D reconstruction in the en face view, respectively. (F) Postclip deployment, hemodynamic assessment demonstrating systolic dominant PV flow on Doppler. ICE, intracardiac echocardiography; MPR, multiplanar reconstruction; TEER, transcatheter edge-to-edge repair.

venous (PV) flow (Fig. 2A–F). As with TEE, real-time imaging is then used to guide clip delivery system (CDS) down to the MV. Assessment of leaflet insertion, residual MR location, and severity are done with similar views with and without color flow Doppler.

Several case reports had demonstrated the safety and feasibility of 3D ICE-guided M-TEER. A recent multicenter registry involving 12 patients who underwent 3D ICE-guided M-TEER demonstrated not only excellent safety and feasibility but also high procedural success as defined by deployment of at least 1 clip with a residual MR of 2+ or less.[9] Several limitations with the use of 3D ICE for M-TEER exist. The crux of M-TEER is high-fidelity imaging confirming leaflet capture and insertion. Given 3D ICE catheter has one-third of the imaging crystals as compared with TEE, which directly affects image quality, it remains uncertain whether 3D ICE could become more adoptable even in patients without contraindication to TEE. There is interest given the perceived benefit of avoiding an imager and/or anesthesia. However, the authors of this article would caution this rationale as conscious sedation-based M-TEER has been performed[10] but patients can often move or have prohibitive tidal volumes that would create unnecessary risk during the procedure. Furthermore, the use of 3D ICE does not avoid

the need for an imager because there still is a significant amount of console manipulation that is done intraprocedurally. Other limitations consist of ability to treat noncentral pathologic condition and/or those with functional MR because much of the published series to date have treated central pathologic condition and/or primary MR.

LEFT ATRIAL APPENDAGE OCCLUSION

In patients with nonvalvular atrial fibrillation at high risk for stroke and bleeding events, transcatheter left atrial appendage closure (LAAO) has been shown to be noninferior with respect to composite points of stroke, cardiovascular death, and bleeding, compared with either warfarin or direct oral anticoagulants. Two current systems are available in the United States. The WATCHMAN FLX device (Boston Scientific, St. Paul, MN), which consists of a self-expanding nitinol alloy frame with a polyethylene tetraphthalate fabric membrane, was the first Food and Drug Administration-approved percutaneous LAAO device and the most extensively studied. Much of the experience with 3D ICE-guided LAAO is with the WATCHMAN FLX system.

As with 3D ICE-guided M-TEER, ultrasound-guided transfemoral access is obtained either in a stacked configuration or via bilateral femoral

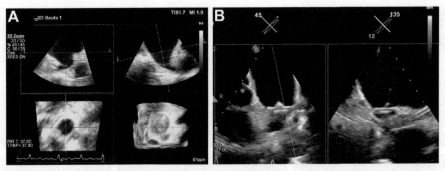

Fig. 3. 3D ICE-guided LAAO. (*A*) MPR with orthogonal views of the LAA and *en face* views with 3D reconstruction. (*B*) X-plane of LAA demonstrating appropriate device sizing and stable position. Color flow Doppler can be applied to assess seal. LAA, left atrial appendage.

venous access. Transeptal puncture is then performed, and either through a floss technique or balloon septostomy, the ICE catheter is advanced into the LA. Once the 3D ICE catheter is advanced into the LA, there are generally 3 "park" positions that the ICE catheter is positioned with further assessment performed via the console. In order of decreasing priority: mid-LA view, mitral view, and pulmonary vein view. In the mid-LA view, the ICE catheter rotated clockwise or counterclockwise until the MV is in view. Posterior flex is then performed until the left atrial appendage (LAA) is in view with further slight adjustments with catheter clockwise/counterclockwise (CW/CCW) and/or left/right knob manipulation. Once the LAA is in view, a series of views are obtained, which can be somewhat analogous to the traditional TEE views (mitral view, aortic view, and pulmonary artery view). The goal of the 0, 45, 90, and 135 planes via TEE is to assess the LAA predeployment and postdeployment in a near 360° fashion. The 3D ICE views noted above achieve the same in similar fashion, although one less view. Once baseline-imaging views are obtained, the LAA delivery sheath is advanced into the LA over the preexisting LA rail wire and the dilator removed. In standard fashion, the 5Fr pigtail catheter is then advanced and directed into the LAA for the traditional appendogram. The device and delivery catheter are then inserted into the LAA and unsheathed with full deployment into the LAA per standard fashion. Compression characteristics are analyzed under 3D ICE. After release criteria are met (position, anchor, size, and seal), the device is detached from the delivery catheter. Final LA appendogram may be performed and the guide and delivery catheter are removed.

As noted above, standard TEE views at 0, 45, 90 and 135° views can be challenging using 3D

ICE due to limited range of catheter motion and different vantage point compared with mid-esophageal TEE views. The incorporation of 3D ICE does allow for *en face* views, providing an excellent visualization and assessment of LAA size and anatomy, assessment of thrombus and ultimately guiding device selection, as well as deployment of device and evaluation for immediate postprocedural complications (**Fig. 3A and B**).

Multiple studies have evaluated the role of 3D ICE for LAAO compared with TEE and have demonstrated similar technical success with no significant difference in major procedural-related events between the 2 groups. Many of these studies have used 2D ICE. Follow-up at 45 days had similar rates of peridevice leak, thrombi, and iatrogenic ASDs.[11,12] The specific role for 3D ICE and whether the added expense leads to better outcomes relative to 2D is under investigation.

TRICUSPID TRANSCATHETER EDGE-TO-EDGE REPAIR

Perhaps, the space with highest potential for 3D ICE utilization is with the emerging field of transcatheter tricuspid valve (TV) interventions. Results from a landmark multicenter, parallel, randomized control trial demonstrated effectiveness in transcatheter edge-to-edge repair with significant improvement in quality of life.[13] Several factors that might make 3D ICE more advantageous than TEE for imaging guidance include the less than robust imaging obtained with TEE due to the suboptimal anterior location and conversely the excellent direct visualization of the TV apparatus and right ventricle with 3D ICE (**Fig. 4 A and B**). Several case reports/series have established a proof of concept for 3D ICE-guided T-TEER

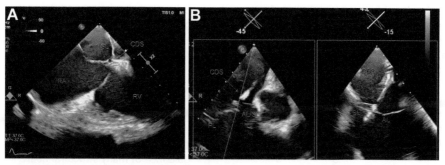

Fig. 4. Tricuspid-TEER with 3D ICE. (*A*) Excellent grasping view of the anterior and septal leaflet in a patient with severely dilated RA/RV and horizontal heart position. (*B*) X-plane with "home view" on left demonstrating mobile posterior leaflet and on the right with clear grasping view of the septal and anterior leaflet. AL, anterior leaflet; CDS, clip delivery system; PL, posterior leaflet; RA, right atrium; RV, right ventricle; SL, septal leaflet.

and more large-scale clinical trials are needed to clarify benefits are ongoing.

TRICUSPID AND MITRAL VALVE-IN-VALVE

As the number of bioprosthetic valve implantation increases, the cases that will require reintervention due to structural deterioration undoubtedly increase. When redo surgery is prohibitive, transcatheter mitral and TV replacement may be an option. Multiple case reports have demonstrated feasibility with 3D ICE guided valve-in-valve under moderate sedation with good recovery, in some instances discharged on the same day.[14,15] Specifically for mitral valve-in-valve, 3D not only is able to help guide transeptal puncture but also through the LA view, direct visualization of the bioprosthetic MV apparatus can help to guide successful deployment (Fig. 5 A and B). As with other structural interventions that typically rely on TEE for periprocedural imaging, 3D ICE is an especially attractive option when general anesthesia is contraindicated or when TEE imaging windows are limited.

PERIVALVULAR LEAK CLOSURE

PVL is not uncommon after valve replacement, occurring in 5% to 17% of patients.[16] In the majority of these cases, these findings are incidentally noted on follow-up imaging and are clinically insignificant. In cases where the PVL is significant, patients can develop signs and symptoms of heart failure. These patients are also at an increased risk for endocarditis and hemolysis, which can lead to profound anemia. Whether the original prosthesis was from a surgical or transcatheter approach, surgical repair is often the preferred approach for closure. However, surgical outcomes vary dramatically and carry high perioperative risks. This is especially true in cases where a transcatheter approach for valve replacement was undertaken due to the prohibitive risks of surgery. As a result, transcatheter PVL closures have become more attractive because they often carry less risk with shorter procedural and recovery times. As with other structural heart procedures, TEE guidance is *sine qua non* for procedural success. Similarly, when TEE is contraindicated, 3D ICE can be considered for

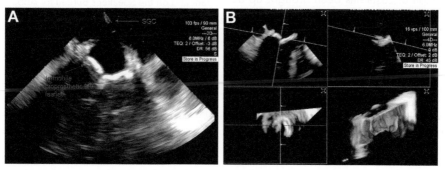

Fig. 5. Mitral valve-in-valve with 3D ICE guidance. (*A*) Direct LA view demonstrating bioprosthetic leaflet thickening with limited leaflet mobility and resultant severe mitral stenosis. (*B*) MPR with *en face* view with and without 3D reconstruction. MV, mitral valve; SGC, steerable guide catheter.

periprocedural guidance with similar degrees of success.

Imaging guidance with 3D ICE is often done from the RA and RV views. The technical aspects of the procedure depend on the valve and the location of the PVL. With periaortic leaks, a retrograde approach via transfemoral access is often preferred. A telescoping catheter system is created, typically a multipurpose or Amplatzer Left guiding catheter along with an angled glide catheter nestled inside. Using a 0.035″ glidewire to cross the defect, the catheter is then advanced over the wire. Once the wire is removed, the vascular plug is then advanced into position and delivered across the defect. Direct LA views can be pursued in cases of peri-mitral leaks because it allows for direct visualization of the prosthesis. An antegrade or retrograde approach for closure depends on the location of the leak. More specifically, leaks along the lateral aspect of the valve, seen in the *en face* view, typically are closed via and antegrade approach from the LA while a retro-grade approach is often preferred if the leak is more septal. In either case, periprocedural 3D ICE imaging aids in device selection and sizing and provides real-time assessment of procedural success, degree of residual leak, and periproce-dural complications.

SUMMARY

A discussion on 3D ICE-guidance for structural heart interventions is not complete without assessing the limitations, of which there are several. Most notable is the lack of operator fa-miliarity and limited consensus from various im-aging societies and organizations on technique and imaging windows. The need for additional vascular access and transseptal puncture or balloon dilatation can contribute to the poten-tial complications of the procedure. Finally, consideration of costs has been brought up as well as to why early adoption and utilization have been limited. This last issue is not as clear, and depending on the cost structure of the or-ganization, the need for anesthesia support and time associated with general anesthesia may offset costs associated with 3D ICE cathe-ters themselves. What is clear is that 3D ICE can be a powerful imaging modality for periproce-dural guidance of many structural heart pro-cedures when TEE is prohibitive. Increasing experience and evidence is still needed to define its role when there are not contraindica-tions to TEE; although, where local practice constraints affect TEE availability, the positive experiences of multiple high-volume centers suggest that 3D ICE may have a role as first-line procedural imaging as imaging quality improves.

CLINICS CARE POINTS

- TEE is the gold standard for intraprocedural guidance of many structural heart interventions
- Patients with contraindications to TEE such as esophageal/gastric disease, cervical/thoracic spinal disease, or coagulopathies, have limited options
- Although there are no guidelines for 3D ICE for structural heart interventions, earlier case reports and case series have demonstrated safety and feasibility for guidance of ASD/PFO closures, mitral and tricuspid TEER, mitral/tricuspid ViV, and PVL closures
- In select cases, imaging guidance with 3D ICE is a viable alternative with a high degree of procedural success
- When no TEE contraindications exist, the role of 3D ICE for guidance of structural interventions remains unclear and more data are needed

ACKNOWLEDGEMENTS

No acknowledgements.

FUNDING

No funding for this project.

DECLARATION OF INTERESTS

The author, Gagan D. Singh, is an Educational Consul-tant and on the Speaker's Bureau for Abbott Structural Heart and Phillips. Dr Pham serves as a consultant for Siemens Healthineers.

REFERENCES

1. Alqahtani F, Bhirud A, Aljohani S, et al. Intra-car-diac versus transesophageal echocardiography to guide transcatheter closure of interatrial communi-cations: nationwide trend and comparative anal-ysis. J Intervent Cardiol 2017;30:234–41.
2. Grewal J, Mankad S, Freeman WK, et al. Real-time three-dimensional transesophageal echocardiog-raphy in the intraoperative assessment of mitral valve disease. J Am Soc Echocardiogr 2009;22:34.

3. Enriquez A, Saenz LC, Rosso R, et al. Use of intracardiac echocardiography in interventional cardiology. Circulation 2018;137:2278–94.

4. Nishimura RA, Otto CM, Bonow RO, et al. AHA/ACC guideline for the management of patients with valvular heart disease: a report of the American College of Cardiology/American Heart Association Task Force on Practice Guidelines. J Am Coll Cardiol 2014;63:e57.

5. Stone GW, Lindenfeld JA, Abraham WT, et al, on behalf of the COAPT Investigators. Transcatheter Mitral-Valve Repair in Patients With Heart Failure. N Engl J Med 2018. https://doi.org/10.1056/NEJMoa1806640.

6. Sorajja P, Ukaigwe AC. Edge-to-edge repair: past challenge, current case selection and future advances. Ann Cardiothorac Surg 2021;10(1):43–9.

7. Yap J, Rogers JH, Aman E, et al. MitraClip Implantation Guided by Volumetric Intracardiac Echocardiography: Technique and Feasibility in Patients Intolerant to Transesophageal Echocardiography. Cardiovasc Revascularization Med 2021;28S:85–8.

8. Sanchez C, Yakubov S, Singh G, et al. 4-Dimensional Intracardiac Echocardiography in Transcatheter Mitral Valve Repair With the Mitraclip System. J Am Coll Cardiol Img 2021;14(10):2033–40.

9. Pham TH, Tso J, Sanchez CE, et al. Volumetric intracardiac echocardiogram-guided MitraClip in patients intolerant to transesophageal echocardiogram: Results from a multicenter registry. JSCAI 2023;6(2):1000046.

10. Patzelt J, Ulrich M, Magunia H, et al. Comparison of deep sedation with general anesthesia in patients undergoing percutaneous mitral valve repair. J Am Heart Assoc 2017;6(12):e007485.

11. Berti S, Pastormerlo LE, Santoro G, et al. Intracardiac Versus Transesophageal Echocardiographic Guidance for Left Atrial Appendage Occlusion: The LAAO Italian Multicenter Registry. JACC Cardiovasc Interv 2018;11(11):1086–92.

12. Alkhouli M, Chaker Z, Alqahtani F, et al. Outcomes of routine intracardiac echocardiography to guide left atrial appendage occlusion. JACC Clin Electrophysiol 2020. https://doi.org/10.1016/j.jacep.2019.11.014.

13. Sorajja P, Whisenant B, Hamid N, et al, on behalf of the TRILUMINATE Pivotal Investigators. Transcatheter repair for patients with tricuspid regurgitation. N Engl J Med 2023;388:1833–42.

14. Hassan A, Alkhouli M, Thaden J, et al. 3D Intracardiac echo-guided transseptal mitral valve-in-valve under conscious sedation. J Am Coll Cardiol Intv 2022;15(9):e103–5.

15. Bhardwaj B, Lantz G, Golwala H, et al. Transcatheter valve-in-valve mitral valve replacement using 4d intracardiac echocardiogram and conscious sedation. Structural Heart 2022;6(3):100046.

16. Hammermeister K, Sethi GK, Henderson WG, et al. Outcomes 15 years after valve replacement with a mechanical versus a bioprosthetic valve: final report of the Veterans Affairs randomized trial. J Am Coll Cardiol 2000;36:1152–8.

Use of Computed Tomography for Left Atrial Appendage Occlusion Procedure Planning and Post-Procedure Assessment

Pankaj Malhotra, MD[a,b,*]

KEYWORDS

- Cardiac computed tomography • LAAO • Transcatheter • Atrial appendage occlusion
- Anticoagulation • Atrial fibrillation • Thromboembolism • Transesophageal echocardiography

---

KEY POINTS

- Transcatheter left atrial appendage occlusion (LAAO) is another approach to deal with systemic anticoagulation in those patients who have non-valvular atrial fibrillation with an increased risk for thromboembolic events.
- Pre- and post-procedural imaging is important for gaining technical success as it allows practitioners to find out contraindications, select relevant devices, and recognize procedural complications.
- Although transesophageal echocardiography has traditionally served as the preeminent imaging modality in LAAO, cardiac computed tomography (CT) imaging has also emerged as a noninvasive surrogate given its excellent isotropic spatial resolution, multiplanar reconstruction capability, rapid temporal resolution, and large field of view.
- This article demonstrates the utility of CT in the analysis of transcatheter LAAO, particularly focusing on pre- and post-intervention.

INTRODUCTION

Transcatheter left atrial appendage occlusion (LAAO) is an alternative to systemic anticoagulation in patients with non-valvular atrial fibrillation with increased risk for thromboembolic events.[1–4] Pre- and post-procedural imaging is essential for technical success, allowing practitioners to identify contraindications, select appropriate devices, and recognize procedural complications. Although transesophageal echocardiography (TEE) has traditionally served as the preeminent imaging modality in LAAO, cardiac computed tomography (CT) imaging has emerged as a noninvasive surrogate given its excellent isotropic spatial resolution, multiplanar reconstruction capability, rapid temporal resolution, and large field of view.[5–8] In this article, we hope to demonstrate the utility of CT in the assessment of transcatheter LAAO, with a particular focus pre- and post-intervention.

TRANSCATHETER LEFT ATRIAL APPENDAGE OCCLUSION DEVICES

Multiple percutaneous left atrial appendage (LAA) closure devices have been developed, including internal LAA plug and external LAA occluder devices. This article focuses on imaging

---

[a] Department of Imaging, Mark Taper Imaging Center, Cedars Sinai Medical Center, 8700 Beverly Boulevard, Taper M335, Los Angeles, CA 90048, USA; [b] Smidt Heart Institute, Cedars Sinai Medical Center, Los Angeles, CA, USA
* Department of Imaging, Mark Taper Imaging Center, Cedars Sinai Medical Center, 8700 Beverly Boulevard, Taper M335, Los Angeles, CA 90048.
E-mail address: Pankaj.Malhotra@cshs.org

Intervent Cardiol Clin 13 (2024) 19–28
https://doi.org/10.1016/j.iccl.2023.08.006
2211-7458/24/© 2023 Elsevier Inc. All rights reserved.

considerations for endocardially placed devices, specifically the Watchman FLX occluder device (Boston Scientific, Natick, MA) and Amplatzer Amulet device (Abbott, Chicago, IL). The Watchman FLX device is anchored by fixation barbs and can accommodate larger or smaller LAA dimensions than the original Watchman.[9–11] Conversely, the Amulet is stabilized by an anchoring lobe with fixation wires and a proximal occluder disk (Fig. 1).[12]

The Watchman FLX device is available in five sizes (20, 24, 27, 31, and 35 mm) and treats LAA ostia ranging from 14 to 32 mm.[11] Amulet device sizes include 16, 18, 20, 22, 25, 28, 31, and 34 mm.[12] Compared with the Watchman FLX, the Amulet device can accommodate both larger and smaller LAA orifices (11–32 mm). In a randomized trial comparing the two devices, the Amulet device was noninferior to the Watchman in terms of primary safety and efficacy endpoints but was associated with more procedure-related complications.[13]

COMPUTED TOMOGRAPHY PROTOCOL

A multidetector CT scanning platform with at least 64 detector rows is necessary for adequate imaging.[14] A uniform CT protocol is used pre-and post-LAAO, though higher tube potential is used in the post-procedural setting to minimize beam-hardening artifacts. Given the variability of LAA size throughout the cardiac cycle and prevalent atrial fibrillation at the time of imaging, retrospective electrocardiographic gating is frequently used.[15] However, in cases of sinus rhythm with slow heart rates or with advanced scanning platforms, some centers may be able to use prospective electrocardiographic triggering to minimize radiation exposure. Either biphasic or triphasic contrast injections are administered to reduce contrast-related streak artifacts. Either a test bolus or bolus tracking method can be used to trigger image acquisition, though bolus tracking may be preferred to reduce repeated contrast exposure to patients and lessen scan times. In doing so, a region of interest is placed in the left atrium (LA) or ascending aorta.[16] Tube potential is set between 80 to 140 kV (based on the patient's body mass index), and images are obtained from the carina to the diaphragm during an expiratory breath-hold. An additional delayed scan is performed 60 seconds after the arterial phase to evaluate for thrombus, an absolute contraindication to LAAO in pre-procedural imaging (Fig. 2).[17,18] Slow flow, conversely, would be expected to resolve on delayed imaging.

Pre-Procedural Assessment

The LAA is a thin-walled, slender outpouching of the anterolateral LA, located in the atrioventricular groove. It is composed of three regions: the ostium (the opening from the LA), the neck, and the body.[19,20] LAAs differ significantly in size, shape, and number of lobes, which impacts LAAO device selection and procedural planning.[21,22] The principal aims of pre-procedural imaging are to assess LAA size and shape for appropriate device selection and recognize pitfalls that may lead to procedural complications. Measurements with TEE are typically smaller than those of CT; the use of TEE alone may exclude up to 23% of patients due to undersizing.[7,21,23] In addition, the use of pre-procedural CT for LAAO is associated with better procedural success and improved procedural efficiency versus TEE—procedures guided by CT demonstrated a lower average number of devices used, fewer guide catheters, shorter procedure times, and lower radiation and contrast material doses.[24,25]

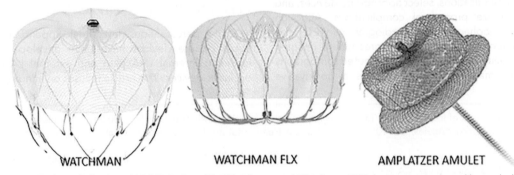

Fig. 1. Endocardially placed LAAO devices. The Watchman and Watchman FLX devices are anchored by occluders with fixation barbs and differ in that the FLX device can accommodate more LAA dimensions. The Amulet device is stabilized by an anchoring lobe and a proximal occluder.

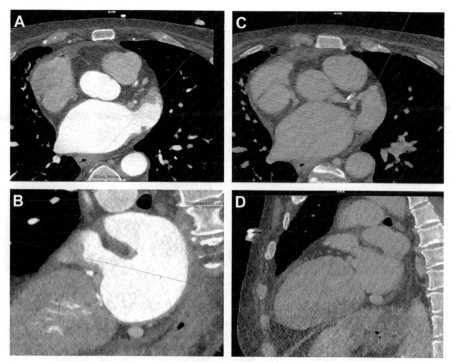

Fig. 2. LAA thrombus assessment. (*A, B*) Multiplanar images immediately following contrast administration demonstrate hypodensities present in the LAA, concerning for thrombus versus slow flow. (*C, D*) Multiplanar delayed images acquired 60 seconds after (*A*) and (*B*), in which there is resolution of the hypodensities. In this case, a diagnosis of slow flow was made (as opposed to thrombus, which would remain present on delayed images).

Left Atrial Appendage Anatomy

Four main types of LAA anatomy have been described: windsock, chicken wing, cauliflower, and cactus (**Fig. 3**).[22,26] The windsock subtype is characterized by a long single dominant lobe and given its simplistic anatomy, allows for the easiest measurement and LAAO device deployment. The cactus type features a dominant central lobe with smaller secondary lobes extending from the central lobe superiorly and inferiorly. Given the presence of a larger central lobe, measurement and device implantation are also usually straightforward in cactus anatomy. The chicken wing subtype is the most common LAA morphology, distinguished by a prominent bend in the proximal or middle portion of the dominant lobe. Although this morphology is associated with the lowest incidence of thromboembolic events, it is considered less optimal for LAAO due to an often short proximal portion.[27] Finally, the cauliflower subtype is the least common type but is also associated with the highest risk of stroke.[26] This type is multilobed, irregular, and typified by a short length relative to the size of the orifice that may not accommodate LAAO.

Left Atrial Appendage Occlusion Device Selection

In addition to assessment of LAA shape, accurate sizing is imperative for successful occlusion. LAA measurements are obtained from the phase with largest dimension using multiplanar reconstruction, achieved with CT given its isotropic voxel construction.[28,29] Device undersizing can lead to embolization and peri-device leaks, whereas oversizing may contribute to device erosion and LAA rupture.

The LAA ostium, LAA length, and device landing zone are the principal elements of LAAO device sizing and deployment. Optimal LAAO device seating is achieved when the atrial end of the device is flush with the plane of the ostium. The landing zone is this location where the device will ideally sit within the confines of the LAA and is defined as the region between the main lobe of the LAA and the course of the left circumflex artery.[7,28] To determine the landing zone, an oblique section is drawn perpendicular to the long axis of the left circumflex in the axial images. In the long axis two-chamber view, the LAA ostium is defined as the plane between the circumflex and the Coumadin ridge. A subsequent *en face*

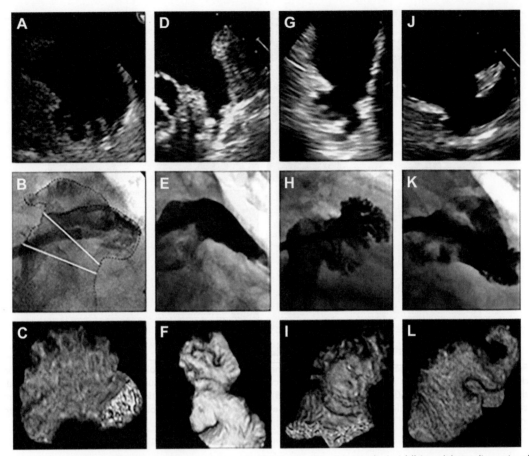

Fig. 3. The four different LAA morphologies as shown by TEE (*top*), cine angiography (*middle*), and three-dimensional computed tomography (*bottom*). Cauliflower (*A–C*), windsock (*D–F*), cactus (*G–I*), and chicken wing (*J–L*).

view is generated at this location for measurements of the maximal and minimal LAA diameters, area, and perimeter, used for device sizing. In the sagittal and coronal views, the length of the LAA is measured from the center of the LAA ostium to the distal tip of the main lobe, dictating the depth necessary for targeted device deployment (Fig. 4). This process also enables practitioners to anticipate intra-procedural C-arm angles and optimal catheter tip positioning.

Each LAAO device has specific sizing instructions and optimal landing zone: the Watchman device uses the maximal LAA diameter with a landing zone 10 to 20 mm inside the LAA from the Coumadin ridge, whereas the Amplatzer Amulet devices use a perimeter-derived diameter with a landing zone ≥10 mm in width with a distal lobe 1.5 to 3.4 mm larger than the landing zone.[28,30]

Relationship to Other Structures
Given its high-resolution images with large field of view, CT imaging is also optimal for the assessment of adjacent anatomical structures, listed below, which may impact procedural success.

Interatrial septum
CT evaluation of the interatrial septum allows for thorough assessment for abnormalities, including atrial septal defects, patent foramen ovale, septal aneurysms, and lipomatous hypertrophy.[31] A pre-existing atrial septal defect or patent foramen ovale should not be used for transseptal access given an increased risk for procedural complications with their use and potential absence of sealing. Lipomatous hypertrophy, conversely, may limit ease of transseptal puncture or increase the likelihood of septal tearing.[32] Thus, the presence of such defects may inform practitioners to consider an alternative location of transseptal puncture rather than the commonly used infero-posterior fossa ovalis.

Coumadin ridge
The Coumadin ridge, located between the LAA and left superior pulmonary vein (LSPV), is typically a narrow structure whose width may affect device sizing. Thinner ridges (≤5 mm) may increase the risk for pulmonary vein impingement with larger devices. Conversely, wider ridges

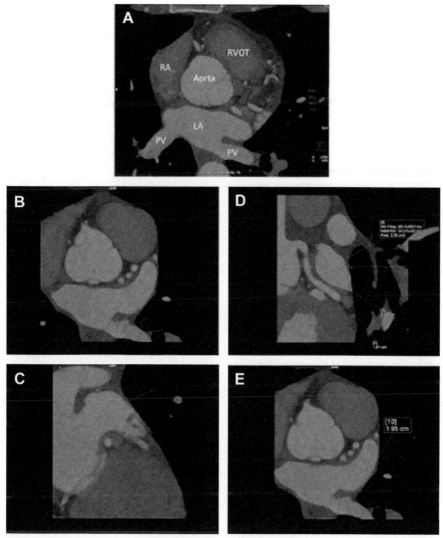

Fig. 4. LAA ostium measurement. (*A*) An axial CT image is used to isolate the left circumflex coronary artery (*red arrow*). (*B, C*) Multiplanar reformatted CT images of the left ventricle and LAA shows the LAA ostium. (*D*) En face view of the LAA ostium, where the maximum diameter, minimum diameter, perimeter, and area are measured. (*E*) From the ostium, the available depth for LAAO device implantation is measured.

(>5 mm) may allow for more flexibility with device oversizing.[29]

Pulmonary veins
Given its proximity to the LAA, the LSPV may be used as a hub for placement of guidewires that support device delivery sheath introduction.[33] Determination of the LAA-LSPV relationship can be performed rapidly with CT imaging, in addition to delineation of complete pulmonary venous anatomy (number of veins, vein sizes/stenoses, and branching patterns).

Optional non-LAA cardiac anatomical considerations may include the evaluation of the pericardium (pericardial effusion), cardiac valves (morphology, calcification, focal thickening) and coronary arteries (ostium, course, branches, calcifications, and stenoses).[15] For instance, CT can clearly delineate the presence of a sinoatrial branch from the left circumflex artery that may course between the LAA and LSPV, which subsequently may influence device sizing.

POST-PROCEDURAL ASSESSMENT

Post-procedurally, patients traditionally continue oral anticoagulation therapy for 45 days after LAAO to allow for device endothelialization. After this time, a TEE is performed to evaluate for procedural or device-related complications, including thrombus or the presence of a significant peri-device leak. Although CT has conventionally been used in patients with equivocal or nondiagnostic TEE findings, technologic advances have improved CT imaging such that it now an alternative for patient evaluation post-LAAO.[34]

Normal Post-Procedural Computed Tomography Imaging

Normally, the LAAO device is well seated in the landing zone between the LA and LAA. The Watchman FLX device should demonstrate 10% to 30% compression compared with the original device size, whereas the Amulet device should have its axis in line with the LAAO neck axis.[35] With a complete seal and device endothelialization, there should be no contrast opacification either around the device or more distally (Fig. 5). It may also be possible to visualize slow flow or thrombus in the LAA distal to the device, though recent studies have shown that complete thrombosis in the device in only seen in 27% of patients at 6 months.[34]

Evaluation of Complications

CT imaging is also optimal for the assessment of procedural complications, listed below.

- Peri-Device Leaks and Incomplete LAAO: The presence of contrast patency in the

LAA post-intervention indicates a peri-device leak (Fig. 6). One analysis quantified that a patent LAA (residual leak) had mean 352.2 ± 136.4 Hounsfield unit (HU) compared with mean 65.2 ± 17.4 HU in occluded LAA (P < .0001). It also noted that all occluded LAA had radiodensity less than 100 HU and contrast opacification less than 25% of the LA.[36] Consequently, in current clinical practice, an LAA is defined as patent if its density is ≥ 100 HU or ≥25% of that of the LA.[37] The location of the leak is identified on CT by the presence of a contrast-enhanced trail adjacent to the device and can be seen in up to 68.5% of patients.[10,38,39] Leaks can be classified as minimal (<1 mm), mild (1–3 mm), moderate (4–5 mm), or severe (>5 mm, also referred to as incomplete closure). Risk factors for peri-device leak development include wide LAA ostium, large landing zone, device undersizing, non-coaxial delivery, or lack of endothelialization. CT is more sensitive than echocardiography for the identification of peri-device leaks; the differential diagnosis for a small defect on CT also includes transfabric leaks or

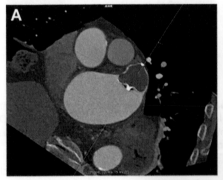
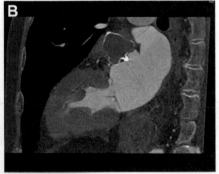
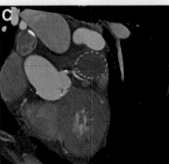

Fig. 5. Well-seated LAAO device on post-procedural CT imaging. In this example, a complete seal and device endothelialization is noted by the lack of contrast opacification either around the device or more distally. Multiplanar reformatted images are shown (*A, B*) in addition to an en face plane (*C*).

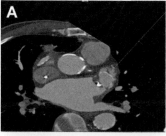
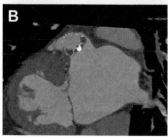
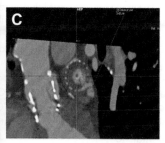

Fig. 6. Peri-LAAO device leak. In this case, there is no complete seal as evidenced by complete contrast opacification of the LAA despite the presence of the occluder device. Multiplanar reformatted images are shown (A, B) in addition to an en face plane (C) illustrating a 4-mm posterolateral gap.

failure of endothelialization.[38,40] Because endothelialization may occur up to 6 months after LAAO, follow-up CT is generally recommended. Recently, even small peri-device leaks less than 5 mm in size with Watchman devices were found to be associated with increased thromboembolism risk, warranting consideration of anticoagulation.[41]

- Device-Related Thrombus: Similarly to pre-LAAO imaging, a thrombus would appear as a hypoattenuating lesion on the surface of the LAAO device that remains present in delayed images.[42] Conversely, slow flow-related defects would be expected to resolve on delayed images. An uncommon complication post-LAAO, device-related thrombus can occur in the setting of incomplete LAAO, high CHA2DS2VASc score for assessment of stroke risk in atrial fibrillation (congestive heart failure, hypertension, age, diabetes, transient ischemic attack/stroke, vascular disease, age greater than 75 years, sex category), or low left ventricular ejection fraction.[34,40] The presence of thrombus portrays an increased risk for thromboembolic events and also may warrant consideration of anticoagulation.

- Device Embolization: A rare complication, embolization is more common in the setting of wide LAA ostium, large landing zone, device undersizing, non-coaxial delivery, and shallow depth of placement.[43] Larger devices typically embolize to the LA or left ventricle, whereas smaller devices may be found in the descending aorta.

- Device Erosion: An extremely rare complication, device erosion through the LAA into the adjacent pulmonary artery, or LSPV can present as cardiac tamponade.[44] It is most commonly associated with device oversizing. CT may help identify the location of the LAAO device as well as the site of erosion/bleeding.

- Pericardial Effusion: Pericardial effusions may occur due to cardiac injury during the transseptal puncture or are related to injury from device deployment.[45] Effusions are commonly seen within 24 hours post-LAAO and are commonly identified during intra-procedural imaging. CT, however, can be useful to distinguish the type of effusion as the presence of high attenuation values may suggest hemopericardium.[45]

SUMMARY

LAAO is an increasingly popular management stratagem to systemic anticoagulation in patients with non-valvular atrial fibrillation. Although TEE has served as the prevailing imaging modality during this structural intervention, CT imaging is an excellent noninvasive alternative for the evaluation of patients undergoing LAAO for both pre-and post-procedural assessments.

CLINICS CARE POINTS

- Computed tomography (CT) imaging is a useful noninvasive surrogate for left atrial appendage occlusion (LAAO) given its excellent isotropic spatial resolution, multiplanar reconstruction capability, rapid temporal resolution, and large field of view.

- In the pre-procedural setting, CT is invaluable in its ability to evaluate the LAA for device selection, including delineation of left atrial appendage (LAA) anatomy, LAA landing zone size, and preferred depth of implantation.

- Pre-procedural CT is also instrumental to identify spatial relationships between the LAA and its adjacent structures, helping practitioners recognize hazards that may lead to procedural complications.

- Post-procedurally, CT clearly defines successful LAAO device positioning and endothelialization.

- CT is readily able to help diagnose procedural complications including peri-device leaks and incomplete LAAO, device-related thrombus, embolization, erosion, and pericardial effusion.

DISCLOSURES

The author has nothing to disclose.

REFERENCES

1. Holmes DR, Reddy VY, Turi ZG, et al. Percutaneous closure of the left atrial appendage versus warfarin therapy for prevention of stroke in patients with atrial fibrillation: a randomised non-inferiority trial. Lancet 2009;374(9689):534–42.

2. Reddy VY, Doshi SK, Sievert H, et al. Percutaneous left atrial appendage closure for stroke prophylaxis in patients with atrial fibrillation: 2.3-Year Follow-up of the PROTECT AF (watchman left atrial appendage system for embolic protection in patients with atrial fibrillation) trial. Circulation 2013; 127(6):720–9.

3. Reddy VY, Sievert H, Halperin J, et al. Percutaneous left atrial appendage closure vs warfarin for atrial fibrillation: a randomized clinical trial. JAMA 2014; 312(19):1988–98.

4. Writing Group M, January CT, Wann LS, et al. 2019 AHA/ACC/HRS focused update of the 2014 AHA/ACC/HRS guideline for the management of patients with atrial fibrillation: A Report of the American College of Cardiology/American Heart Association Task Force on Clinical Practice Guidelines and the Heart Rhythm Society. Heart Rhythm 2019;16(8):e66–93.

5. Lockwood SM, Alison JF, Obeyesekere MN, et al. Imaging the left atrial appendage prior to, during, and after occlusion. JACC Cardiovasc Imaging 2011;4(3):303–6.

6. Mraz T, Neuzil P, Mandysova E, et al. Role of echocardiography in percutaneous occlusion of the left atrial appendage. Echocardiography 2007;24(4): 401–4.

7. Wang DD, Eng M, Kupsky D, et al. Application of 3-Dimensional Computed Tomographic Image Guidance to WATCHMAN Implantation and Impact on Early Operator Learning Curve: Single-Center Experience. JACC Cardiovasc Interv 2016;9(22): 2329–40.

8. Chue CD, de Giovanni J, Steeds RP. The role of echocardiography in percutaneous left atrial appendage occlusion. Eur J Echocardiogr 2011; 12(10):i3–10.

9. Holmes DR Jr, Reddy VY, Gordon NT, et al. Long-Term Safety and Efficacy in Continued Access Left Atrial Appendage Closure Registries. J Am Coll Cardiol 2019;74(23):2878–89.

10. Reddy VY, Doshi SK, Kar S, et al. 5-Year Outcomes After Left Atrial Appendage Closure: From the PREVAIL and PROTECT AF Trials. J Am Coll Cardiol 2017;70(24):2964–75.

11. Kar S, Doshi SK, Sadhu A, et al. Primary Outcome Evaluation of a Next-Generation Left Atrial Appendage Closure Device: Results From the PINNACLE FLX Trial. Circulation 2021;143(18): 1754–62.

12. Lakkireddy D, Windecker S, Thaler D, et al. Rationale and design for AMPLATZER Amulet Left Atrial Appendage Occluder IDE randomized controlled trial (Amulet IDE Trial). Am Heart J 2019;211:45–53.

13. Lakkireddy D, Thaler D, Ellis CR, et al. Amplatzer Amulet Left Atrial Appendage Occluder Versus Watchman Device for Stroke Prophylaxis (Amulet IDE): A Randomized, Controlled Trial. Circulation 2021;144(19):1543–52.

14. Rajiah P, Alkhouli M, Thaden J, et al. Pre- and Post-procedural CT of Transcatheter Left Atrial Appendage Closure Devices. Radiographics 2021; 41(3):680–98.

15. Korsholm K, Berti S, Iriart X, et al. Expert recommendations on cardiac computed tomography for planning transcatheter left atrial appendage occlusion. JACC Cardiovasc Interv 2020;13(3):277–92.

16. Kaafarani M, Saw J, Daniels M, et al. Role of CT imaging in left atrial appendage occlusion for the WATCHMAN device. Cardiovasc Diagn Ther 2020;10(1):45–58.

17. Hur J, Kim YJ, Lee HJ, et al. Dual-enhanced cardiac CT for detection of left atrial appendage thrombus

in patients with stroke: a prospective comparison study with transesophageal echocardiography. Stroke 2011;42(9):2471–7.

18. Romero J, Cao JJ, Garcia MJ, et al. Cardiac imaging for assessment of left atrial appendage stasis and thrombosis. Nat Rev Cardiol 2014;11(8):470–80.

19. Naksuk N, Padmanabhan D, Yogeswaran V, et al. Left Atrial Appendage: Embryology, Anatomy, Physiology, Arrhythmia and Therapeutic Intervention. JACC Clin Electrophysiol 2016;2(4):403–12.

20. Veinot JP, Harrity PJ, Gentile F, et al. Anatomy of the normal left atrial appendage: a quantitative study of age-related changes in 500 autopsy hearts: implications for echocardiographic examination. Circulation 1997;96(9):3112–5.

21. Nucifora G, Faletra FF, Regoli F, et al. Evaluation of the left atrial appendage with real-time 3-dimensional transesophageal echocardiography: implications for catheter-based left atrial appendage closure. Circ Cardiovasc Imaging 2011;4(5):514–23.

22. Beigel R, Wunderlich NC, Ho SY, et al. The left atrial appendage: anatomy, function, and noninvasive evaluation. JACC Cardiovasc Imaging 2014; 7(12):1251–65.

23. Saw J, Fahmy P, Spencer R, et al. Comparing Measurements of CT Angiography, TEE, and Fluoroscopy of the Left Atrial Appendage for Percutaneous Closure. J Cardiovasc Electrophysiol 2016;27(4):414–22.

24. Eng MH, Wang DD, Greenbaum AB, et al. Prospective, randomized comparison of 3-dimensional computed tomography guidance versus TEE data for left atrial appendage occlusion (PRO3DLAAO). Catheter Cardiovasc Interv 2018; 92(2):401–7.

25. Reddy VY, Holmes D, Doshi SK, et al. Safety of percutaneous left atrial appendage closure: results from the Watchman Left Atrial Appendage System for Embolic Protection in Patients with AF (PROTECT AF) clinical trial and the Continued Access Registry. Circulation 2011;123(4):417–24.

26. Di Biase L, Santangeli P, Anselmino M, et al. Does the left atrial appendage morphology correlate with the risk of stroke in patients with atrial fibrillation? Results from a multicenter study. J Am Coll Cardiol 2012;60(6):531–8.

27. Lupercio F, Carlos Ruiz J, Briceno DF, et al. Left atrial appendage morphology assessment for risk stratification of embolic stroke in patients with atrial fibrillation: A meta-analysis. Heart Rhythm 2016;13(7):1402–9.

28. Vainrib AF, Harb SC, Jaber W, et al. Left Atrial Appendage Occlusion/Exclusion: Procedural Image Guidance with Transesophageal Echocardiography. J Am Soc Echocardiogr 2018;31(4):454–74.

29. Wang Y, Di Biase L, Horton RP, et al. Left atrial appendage studied by computed tomography to help planning for appendage closure device placement. J Cardiovasc Electrophysiol 2010;21(9): 973–82.

30. Cabrera JA, Ho SY, Climent V, et al. The architecture of the left lateral atrial wall: a particular anatomic region with implications for ablation of atrial fibrillation. Eur Heart J 2008;29(3):356–62.

31. Rajiah P, Kanne JP. Computed tomography of septal defects. J Cardiovasc Comput Tomogr 2010;4(4):231–45.

32. Alkhouli M, Rihal CS, Holmes DR Jr. Transseptal Techniques for Emerging Structural Heart Interventions. JACC Cardiovasc Interv Dec 26 2016;9(24): 2465–80.

33. Lindner S, Behnes M, Wenke A, et al. Relation of left atrial appendage closure devices to topographic neighboring structures using standardized imaging by cardiac computed tomography angiography. Clin Cardiol 2019;42(2):264–9.

34. Dieker W, Behnes M, Fastner C, et al. Impact of left atrial appendage morphology on thrombus formation after successful left atrial appendage occlusion: Assessment with cardiac-computed-tomography. Sci Rep 2018;8(1):1670.

35. Behnes M, Akin I, Sartorius B, et al. –LAA Occluder View for post-implantation Evaluation (LOVE)–standardized imaging proposal evaluating implanted left atrial appendage occlusion devices by cardiac computed tomography. BMC Med Imaging 2016; 16:25.

36. Saw J, Fahmy P, DeJong P, et al. Cardiac CT angiography for device surveillance after endovascular left atrial appendage closure. Eur Heart J Cardiovasc Imaging 2015;16(11):1198–206.

37. Galea R, De Marco F, Meneveau N, et al. Amulet or Watchman Device for Percutaneous Left Atrial Appendage Closure: Primary Results of the SWISS-APERO Randomized Clinical Trial. Circulation 2022;145(10):724–38.

38. Lindner S, Behnes M, Wenke A, et al. Assessment of peri-device leaks after interventional left atrial appendage closure using standardized imaging by cardiac computed tomography angiography. Int J Cardiovasc Imaging 2019;35(4):725–31.

39. Sahore A, Della Rocca DG, Anannab A, et al. Clinical Implications and Management Strategies for Left Atrial Appendage Leaks. Card Electrophysiol Clin 2020;12(1):89–96.

40. Alkhouli M, Busu T, Shah K, et al. Incidence and Clinical Impact of Device-Related Thrombus Following Percutaneous Left Atrial Appendage Occlusion: A Meta-Analysis. JACC Clin Electrophysiol 2018;4(12):1629–37.

41. Dukkipati SR, Holmes DR Jr, Doshi SK, et al. Impact of Peridevice Leak on 5-Year Outcomes After Left Atrial Appendage Closure. J Am Coll Cardiol 2022;80(5):469–83.

42. Romero J, Husain SA, Kelesidis I, et al. Detection of left atrial appendage thrombus by cardiac computed tomography in patients with atrial fibrillation: a meta-analysis. Circ Cardiovasc Imaging 2013;6(2):185–94.

43. Alkhouli M, Sievert H, Rihal CS. Device Embolization in Structural Heart Interventions: Incidence, Outcomes, and Retrieval Techniques. JACC Cardiovasc Interv 2019;12(2):113–26.

44. Sepahpour A, Ng MK, Storey P, et al. Death from pulmonary artery erosion complicating implantation of percutaneous left atrial appendage occlusion device. Heart Rhythm 2013;10(12):1810–1.

45. Wilkins B, Fukutomi M, De Backer O, et al. Left Atrial Appendage Closure: Prevention and Management of Periprocedural and Postprocedural Complications. Card Electrophysiol Clin 2020; 12(1):67–75.

The Interventional Imager
How Do We Train the Next Interventional Imagers?

Bashaer Gheyath, MD[a], Edward Chau, MD[b],
Syed Latif, MD[c,1], Thomas W. Smith, MD[b,*]

KEYWORDS

• Interventional imaging • Echocardiography • Cardiovascular computed tomography
• Structural heart disease • Percutaneous treatment of structural heart disease

KEY POINTS

• Percutaneous procedures for structural heart disease are rapidly expanding.
• Increase in percutaneous procedures has led to a heightened need for specialized imagers with targeted training.
• Cardiovascular imagers are an integral part of the multidisciplinary heart team.
• Current reimbursement models may be dissuading physicians from pursuing further specialization in cardiovascular imaging.

INTRODUCTION

In 2011, the first transcatheter aortic valve replacement (TAVR) was approved for symptomatic severe aortic stenosis in patients of prohibitive surgical risk. New device approvals and stepwise label expansions followed. TAVR became an alternative to surgery in low surgical risk patients and even those with degenerated surgically implanted bioprosthetic valves by 2019.[1] At that time, TAVRs exceeded surgical aortic valve replacements in the United States.[2] Extending the indications resulted in rising procedural volumes and expansion of services to more than 500 institutions.[3] By 2026, the number of TAVRs performed is expected to exceed 130,000 annually.[4]

Similarly, mitral valve disease is highly prevalent. Approximately 10,000 transcatheter mitral valve repairs are performed yearly to treat patients with severe, symptomatic mitral regurgitation.[4] Advancements in transcatheter valve therapies led to the emergence of transcatheter edge-to-edge repair (TEER) for tricuspid valve regurgitation with mortality and heart failure hospitalization rates similar to surgical replacement/repair.[5–7] Pulmonic valve transcatheter therapies had been more common in the congenital population; however, this has been steadily increasing to several thousand performed worldwide with trends adopted by adult interventional cardiologists.[8,9] These therapies have provided nonsurgical therapeutic options, which are especially appealing to an aging population with multiple comorbidities. The significant growth in TEER and TAVR created an additional need for advanced imaging specialists with expertise in diagnostic multidetector computed tomography (MDCT) but also procedural echocardiography guidance.

[a] Department of Imaging, Cedars Sinai Medical Center, 8700 Beverly Boulevard, Taper, A238, Los Angeles, CA 90048, USA; [b] Division of Cardiovascular Medicine, University of California Davis Medical Center, 4680 Y Street, Suite 2820, Sacramento, CA 95817, USA; [c] Heart and Vascular Institute, Sutter Medical Center, Sacramento, CA, USA

[1] Present address: 8100 Chestnut Court, Granite Bay, CA 95746.
* Corresponding author. 4860 Y Street, Suite 2820 Sacramento, CA 95817.
E-mail address: twrsmith@ucdavis.edu
Twitter: @bgheyath (B.G.)

Intervent Cardiol Clin 13 (2024) 29–38
https://doi.org/10.1016/j.iccl.2023.08.007
2211-7458/24/© 2023 Elsevier Inc. All rights reserved.

Percutaneous procedures extend beyond valve therapies. In patients with secundum atrial septal defect (ASD), percutaneous closure is a safe alternative to surgery when the defect's anatomic characteristics are amenable to the available devices.[10,11] Congenital heart disease guidelines recommend echocardiographic guidance in all percutaneous closures.[12] Guidance may use intracardiac echocardiography (ICE) or transesophageal echocardiography (TEE). TEE is known to be superior to transthoracic echocardiography for imaging the interatrial septum and estimates ASD size just as well as direct measurement during surgery.[13,14]

Other percutaneous devices that require a transseptal puncture include left atrial appendage (LAA) occlusion devices. More than 60 years ago, surgical removal/ligation was the only available approach with increased stroke risks and rates of incomplete exclusion.[15] However, within the last 2 decades, increasingly minimally invasive approaches became available, with multiple percutaneous LAA occlusion options.[16–19] These devices were shown to be non-inferior to oral anticoagulants in the prevention of cardiovascular, neurologic, and bleeding events in high risk patients with atrial fibrillation.[20]

INCREASING NEED FOR INTERVENTIONAL IMAGERS

This growth of transcatheter structural heart interventions has therefore increased the demand for physicians with a specific understanding of anatomy. They require intra-procedural-based and advanced multimodality cardiac imaging training. Interventional cardiac imagers are specialized physicians who possess advanced knowledge and expertise in imaging techniques, anatomy, and pathology specific to interventional cardiovascular procedures. Specifically, they are an integral part of the multidisciplinary heart team (MDHT), which aims to form a consensus on treatment options and procedural approach in a complex patient population. In addition, they are crucial in identifying and reducing intra-procedural complications.[21]

As the aging population grows, the demand for minimally invasive therapeutic options will increase. The number of percutaneous devices and types of interventions will continue to expand and evolve. As these procedures become more complex, there will be a need for ongoing medical education in interventional imaging and further specialized imagers. A skilled interventional cardiac imager is critical

to the growth and success of any high-volume structural heart disease (SHD) program.

MDCT has emerged as a pivotal tool in the planning and guidance of percutaneous structural heart procedures. Its role is most crucial in the pre-procedural planning, device selection, and post-procedural surveillance in patients receiving transcatheter valve therapies and percutaneous LAA closure procedures.

ROLE OF MULTIDETECTOR COMPUTED TOMOGRAPHY IN TRANSCATHETER AORTIC VALVE REPLACEMENT

The evaluation of a patient for TAVR is a complex and multifactorial process. MDCT has high spatial resolution and thus became the standard pre-procedural imaging method in patients undergoing TAVR.[22,23]

Currently available devices fall into two categories: balloon-expandable or self-expandable valves. These differ in physical properties and post-procedural morphology of the newly implanted valve. Therefore, sizing algorithms are not interchangeable between the two valve categories.[24] MDCT helps delineate which valve category may be preferable; for example, in an extremely oval-shaped annulus, a self-expandable valve is preferred. Conversely, in the presence of a dilated ascending aorta (>43 mm) or severely angulated aorta (aortoventricular angle >70°), the preferred valve is a balloon expandable valve.[25]

Pre-TAVR MDCT aims to provide motion-free high-quality images of the aortic valve and root combined with a window range that covers the entire aortic course between the proximal supra-aortic vessels and the ilio-femoral axes for access evaluation.[26]

Many of these devices have different potential access routes and choice of delivery systems. If vascular access difficulties are anticipated, then different valves (eg, SAPIEN valve from Edwards LifeSciences, Irvine, CA) may have the option of a non-femoral approach, bypassing heavily calcified or tortuous/stenotic native arteries.[27] Finally, assessment of the aortic root should include a description of the aortic valve morphology, minimum distance to the coronary artery ostia, and measurement of different annular dimensions at different cross-sectional levels of the sinus. Exact measurements provided by MDCT influence the choice of valve size. Furthermore, MDCT is the modality of choice for valve-in-valve procedure as the size of the in situ surgical aortic valve prosthesis determines the maximum valve size that can be implanted. If the already implanted valve size is not known, this can be deduced from the CT appearance and known standardized measurements.[28,29]

MDCT has largely replaced TEE for TAVR pre-procedural planning.[23] However, in cases with short distances between the aortic annulus and coronary ostia, TEE is more suitable to guide an emerging technique (BASILICA) to avoid coronary obstruction during TAVR. In addition to traditional fluoroscopic guidance, 4D TEE with Multivue and transillumination (TrueVue) rendering capabilities (Philips Healthcare, Amsterdam, the Netherlands) can be complementary for procedural guidance and in pinpointing the location of leaflet laceration.[30,31]

Post-procedurally, MDCT can be used for surveillance of complications. Leaflet thrombosis (which may occur weeks, months, or years post-TAVR) can be seen as hypoattenuated leaflet thickening (HALT). HALT prevalence ranges from 4% to 40% of the post-TAVR population. This has sensitive clinical implications and requires the initiation/intensification of anticoagulation in the post-TAVR population.[32,33]

ROLE OF MULTIDETECTOR COMPUTED TOMOGRAPHY IN PERCUTANEOUS LEFT ATRIAL APPENDAGE CLOSURE

Percutaneous LAA closure is a procedure that benefits from a multimodality imaging approach with MDCT and TEE. LAA anatomy is most commonly classified into four: chicken-wing (~48%; with a significant bend), windsock (~19%; single dominant lobe without a bend), cactus (~30%; dominant lobe with multiple small lobes), and cauliflower (~3%; short and branches into several lobes).[34] LAA shape can increase the technical difficulty for percutaneous closure. Consequently, imaging is essential for preoperative planning, which ranges from equipment selection to implantation strategy to device surveillance post-implantation.[34]

Pre-procedure imaging focuses on excluding LAA thrombus, describing LAA anatomy, measuring LAA dimensions, selecting fluoroscopic angles, and determining sheath selection. TEE is the traditional gold-standard; however, there are several advantages with MDCT, including superior spatial resolution, detailed three-dimensional characterization of LAA anatomy, accurate sizing, and noninvasive image acquisition. In addition, with TEE alone, detecting any anatomic exclusions on the table would lead to case cancellation affecting general anesthesia and catheterization laboratory resources and time.[35] Besides being convenient, MDCT

has also made significant advances with protocol adaptations that can yield positive predictive values and specificities greater than 90% and negative predictive values and sensitivities close to 100% for LAA thrombus detection.[36]

When it comes to describing the LAA, oblique multiplanar reconstructions (MPRs) and 3D volume-rendered images on MDCT should be visualized to establish implant location. MPR images also allow visualization of adjacent structures (such as the left upper pulmonary vein or mitral annulus), which may encounter certain LAA occlusion devices. The angulation of the neck of LAA can be easily determined from coronal and sagittal planes and can assist with sheath selection and anticipated location of a transseptal puncture.[35] Different LAA devices have their own relevant measurements. Specific manufacturer instructions should be adhered to. MDCT measurements should be made at the cardiac phase with the largest LAA dimensions, usually at late atrial diastole (30%–40% of the RR interval).[37] Using MPR, different planes are obtained but the orthogonal "en face" double-oblique view is essential to measure the maximum and minimum dimensions of the LAA ostium. LA depth is also assessed, which may require maximal intensity projections to visualize the entire body of the LAA given its angulations. With regard to TEE measurements, both the LAA orifice and depth must be measured in a minimum of four angles (0°, 45°, 90°, and 135°) and in end-systole (largest LAA dimension). Three-dimensional-TEE may help facilitate assessment of the shape, mean, maximum, and minimum dimension measurements of the LAA. This is especially helpful for highly elliptical LAAs.[38–41]

Intra-procedurally, fluoroscopy and TEE are preferred for LAA closure imaging. ICE is now gaining popularity (and the standard in some centers). The aim is to confirm the lack of thrombus and sizing measurements. Echocardiography has an advantage of live imaging and hemodynamic assessment in different volume loading conditions, which affects LAA sizing. TEE or ICE can provide live imaging of the transseptal needle and sheath position in relation to the fossa ovalis during transseptal puncture. The TEE bicaval (superoinferior) and short-axis (anteroposterior) views of the atrial septum are essential to guide inferior-posterior transseptal punctures. Before device release, it is crucial to interrogate the device in the above-mentioned four angles to ensure appropriate compression, insignificant peri-device leak (<3 mm), and stable tug tests.[35]

Post-procedurally, device surveillance with either TEE or MDCT is recommended following 6 to 12 weeks post-closure. This is primarily for the assessment of device-related thrombus and peri-device leak. The device-related thrombus has been reported to be around 2% to 4% and can be detected on either modality. MDCT has the advantage of assessing the mechanism of residual leaks, differentiating from leaking through the fabric (incomplete endocardialization) or peri-device leak (due to ostial LAA spaces or incomplete seal/off-axis device).[42,43]

WHAT ROLE DOES A COMPREHENSIVE IMAGER PLAY IN THE HEART TEAM?

With the expansion of structural heart procedures to include not only different procedures but also different approaches to the same type of procedure, a structural imager must have a comprehensive understanding of each patient's unique anatomic complexity paired with the growing procedural options. Within the MDHT, the interventional imaging provider has the unique training and expertise to suggest and interpret the diagnostic studies necessary to understand the subtleties of the disease process and assess for procedural access options and potential complications. Armed with that information, the interventional imager can also lead the discussion for procedural imaging options as the diagnostic assessment should provide enough information to determine if TEE will be adequate or if alternative imaging modalities such as TTE or ICE will be necessary to ensure a safe and effective procedure. In patient follow-up, the structural imager should be involved in patient assessment and critically appraise the imaging results and choice of techniques to assess procedural outcome. An interventional imager trained in MDCT, TEE, TTE, and ICE brings a unique perspective to the heart team allowing a comprehensive evaluation of the patient's disease process and the visualization options available to image and guide the structural interventions and follow-up.

THE IMPORTANCE OF TRAINING AND WORKING WITHIN 3D VOLUMES

Not all interventional imagers have undergone post-fellowship training. Many demonstrated an aptitude and interest in imaging during their general fellowship that carried on into their practice. One consistent skill that is apparent in successful imagers is the ability to work within 3D volumes. Current imaging modalities all have the capacity to capture 3D volumes that can then be manipulated either in real-time or post-processing. This similarity creates sufficient overlap such that what one learns in one modality translates to the others. The most accessible modality is MDCT. The cardiac-gated MDCT scans create a very realistic volume to work within, allowing the provider to train their minds to see cardiac structures and their relationships from different views. Once the larger volumes of MDCT are mastered, it becomes very easy to apply those same 3D volume perspectives to smaller fields of view of TTE, TEE, or ICE.

CURRENT IMAGING TRAINING PROGRAMS

In recognizing the growing field of structural cardiology, many centers have developed formal advanced imaging fellowship pathways for trainees to master procedural-based skills and advanced cardiac imaging modalities. However, there is wide variation among training programs due to program-specific resources, procedural volumes, and departmental agreements among cardiology, anesthesiology, and radiology. Some imaging programs may be more heavily radiology-focused with most of the year reading MDCT and cardiac magnetic resonance (CMR) studies that touch other domains of cardiology, such as preventative cardiology and congenital heart disease, in addition to the structurally related cases. There may be little time for hands-on TEE prescreening and intra-procedural experience of structural cases. Other programs may lean more heavily on the advanced echocardiography side with most of the time focused on developing proficiency using the probe in and out of the operating room or catheterization laboratory.

High-volume centers may develop a comprehensive advanced imaging fellowship spanning 2 years that splits time for 1 year focused on MDCT and CMR and the second focused on structural echocardiography. These programs generally heavily encourage and support research through the years. Other programs may have space to train multiple advanced fellows along separate but oftentimes overlapping pathways across 1 year in a hybrid approach. For example, an institution may have an advanced fellow primarily focused on MDCT/CMR training and a second fellow focused on advanced echocardiography. This approach yields several benefits including institutional flexibility with personnel in cases, joint and collaborative learning environments between the trainees, and a shortened training time frame. Most trainees will begin their respective job search early in their ultimate year of training. If they know the type of clinical practice and responsibilities expected of them early on, they may be able to tailor their learning experience more easily in such a hybrid-structured advanced imaging program. Many programs will offer 1-year advanced multimodality training in all four modalities. Although the exposure and teaching capabilities are available, there is generally a focused gravitation toward two of the four modalities to fill in gaps in imaging training during general cardiology fellowship.

VOLUMES REQUIRED IN EACH MODALITY: HOW BEST TO ACHIEVE

The journey of learning through general fellowship is guided by the Core Cardiology Training Symposium (COCATS) training standards that outline progressive skill levels in different cardiovascular arenas.[44] Noninvasive imaging techniques are a key component of evaluating patients with cardiovascular disease. Formal integration of echocardiographic, nuclear, MDCT, and possibly CMR training have become a core component of the general cardiology fellow's curriculum. As such, graduating general cardiologists may be able to highlight their competency as a noninvasive multimodality cardiac imaging specialist by achieving COCATS Level II competencies in selected areas during the standard 3-year general cardiology fellowship.

Although approximately 6 months during the standard 3-year fellowship could be devoted to advanced training, Level III training in general cannot be fully attained in the 3-year general cardiology fellowship and additional time and exposure is needed to achieve respective competencies, including in echocardiography and MDCT. There is wide heterogeneity in the institutional breadth of structural cases and procedures that may be offered to trainees. To unify competencies and expectations of the independent interventional imager, recent expert consensus curricular guidelines by the American Society of Echocardiography (ASE) on interventional echocardiography (IE) and leaders in MDCT SHD imaging, respectively, were developed to highlight training structural imaging competencies.[45–47]

The newly developed Level III-IE designation does not significantly differ from traditional level III echocardiography competencies but places an emphasis on SHD procedures. The ASE writing group recommends an additional 9 to 12 months of advanced echocardiography training in IE irrespective of whether level II or III is achieved in general cardiology fellowship.[45] Similarly, the expert consensus statement for MDCT imaging in SHD interventions recommends an additional 6 to 12 months after cardiology or radiology training with an established SHD cardiac MDCT training program.[47] The minimum recommended case load is described in Table 1.

PROCEDURAL IMAGING TRAINING IN GENERAL FELLOWSHIP

General cardiology trainees interested in interventional imaging need to understand the knowledge and skillsets that will make them valuable team members to the MDHT team. With this understanding, trainees may pursue institutions with adequate volumes to support their interest. While interviewing, they should inquire about the volume and exposure of structural heart interventions and the role that a general fellow may have during their training at that institution. Their exploration of SHD may be limited, however, if the internal medicine graduate did not train at a recognized SHD center. Like how a general fellow pursuing interventional cardiology will need to consider further advanced training in structural heart, chronic total occlusion, or peripheral interventions during their tenure, the multimodality imaging inclined general fellow will need to consider whether they want to pursue interventional imaging.

This decision does not come easy. Additional training comes at a personal, temporal, and financial opportunity cost with sacrifices that each trainee must weigh. Engaging with institutional or national structural imaging or recent graduates will be helpful to understand the landscape of the field better and hopefully aid in making a well-informed decision. Once the decision has been made, most fellows will be exploring advanced imaging programs to pursue further training. The American College of Cardiology has an Advanced Imaging Training Program database that provides insight to different programs based on geography. However, with the growing structural departments nationally, there will be even more non-ACGME accredited advanced imaging fellowships. Proactive trainees will seek those opportunities through informal means, that is, asking for guidance from fellowship mentors in the structural imaging field, emailing structural departmental leaders at prospective institutions, or social media platforms. Many advanced imaging programs are not formally accredited and

Table 1 Minimal recommended procedural volume for advanced echocardiography and cardiac computed tomography in structural heart disease					
Little et al,[45] 2023 (Echo-ASE)		**Wang et al,[54] 2018 (Echo)**		**Leipsic et al,[46] 2019 (CCT)**	
Valvular	30	TAVR	30 (5 ViV)	TAVR	100 (10 aortic ViV)
		MitraClip	25		
		PMBV	10		
		TMVR	5	TMVR	25
		ASD/PFO closure	5	ASD/PFO closure	5
		PVL	5 aortic 5 mitral	PVL	5 aortic 5 mitral
LAAC	10	LAAC	25	LAAC	25
Alcohol septal ablation	10				
ICE	10				

Abbreviations: ASD, atrial septal defect; CCT, cardiac computed tomography; ICE, intracardiac echocardiography; LAAC, left atrial appendage closure; PFO, patent foramen ovale; PMBV, percutaneous mitral balloon valvuloplasty; PVL, paravalvular leak; TAVR, transcatheter aortic valve replacement; TMVR, transcatheter mitral valve replacement.
   Data from Refs.[45,46,54]

federally funded, so there may be gaps in available positions year-to-year, presenting an additional challenge.

Within general cardiology fellowship, the academic schedule should shift toward a career in interventional imaging. Most programs have the flexibility of about 6 months of elective time that can be dedicated to structural imaging. This time should be used to develop or strengthen foundational knowledge in echocardiography or MDCT. Demonstrating special competence through the National Board of Echocardiography ASCeXAM at the beginning of the final year in fellowship is recommended. With the advances in structural imaging guidelines over the last few years, the competency examination has begun highlighting the evaluation of transcatheter valves and their procedural complications. The hands-on experience of performing and interpreting TTE and TEE imaging in SHD will be amplified and solidified after having passed this examination. Time should be spent in the operating room or catheterization laboratory during live cases with SHD faculty learning how to manipulate the probe and knobs. More importantly, exposure to the two-way communication between the interventional imager and structural interventionalist is invaluable.

Training in MDCT is often more limited compared with echocardiography and nuclear exposure despite its increasing role particularly in the evaluation of chest pain and SHD. In a recent survey of cardiology and radiology trainee or early career physicians regarding by Madan and colleagues, although 61% stated that MDCT is or was a part of the core curriculum at their institution, most of that training was in the form of Web-based learning modules or formal lectures.[48] MDCT may be combined with nuclear training under an imaging-specific elective rotation in some programs. With greater emphasis on this modality, some experts have reimagined the MDCT curriculum in general cardiology fellowship and recommend 2 months of dedicated cardiac MDCT time for COCATS Level I competency and 4 months of dedicated time for COCATS Level II competency.[49] Although it may not be necessary or feasible to obtain the Certification of Cardiovascular Computed Tomography during general fellowship, especially if already pursuing an advanced imaging fellowship, delving into the physics, acquisition, and interpretation of this modality will aid in troubleshooting image quality issues and prepare the trainee for advanced training.

Pre-procedural MDHT meetings should concurrently be attended as they provide an opportunity to learn not only the indications and considerations for a particular structural procedure but also how multimodality imaging tools help guide decision-making. Beyond what is available at the training institution, industry partners or national/local structural conferences may have virtual or live practical sessions, device-specific courses, and simulator training workshops for learners that help develop a theoretic and basic understanding of structural cases. These avenues do not supplant the experience derived by being in actual cases where clinical information and imaging findings are integrated and used for critical decisions.

Although every general fellowship has their own strengths and weaknesses, most will have sufficient elective time for the aspiring interventional imager to take advantage of existing strengths within the program. Foundational knowledge in echocardiography, nuclear, and MDCT is essential for the noninvasive cardiologist, but additional time may be possibly carved out for SHD focused imaging. Using these imaging modalities to "see" SHD pathologies provides the competency to apply them across developing structural procedures.

POST-FELLOWSHIP CHALLENGES

In the real-world practice, the opportunity to participate in the development of SHD programs outside of an academic setting continues to grow. However, there are significant challenges mostly in the financial support of advanced imagers.[50] In the United States, most of the physicians are reimbursed according to the "work relative value units" (wRVU) model that was developed by the Centers for Medicare and Medicaid.[51] The premise of this model is that for each work-related task that a physician performs, there is a universal weighted value based on the type of work the physician is performing.[51] For example, a routine TEE has a wRVU of 2.30 (CPT code 93312). A structural heart TEE carries a wRVU value of 4.66 (CPT code 93355). On the surface, this seems to compensate for the increased level of complexity involved in procedural imaging as compared with routine TEEs. However, this does not consider the amount of time required to complete these procedures. A transcatheter mitral valve repair procedure can take up to 3 hours.[52] In that same time, an experienced general cardiologist can see anywhere from 3 to 9 outpatient follow-up visits (using CPT code 99214, this would be a total wRVU of 5.76 for 3 outpatient visits to 17.28 wRVUs for 9 outpatient clinic visits) in an outpatient clinic or interpret 15 TTE studies, which would translate to 21.9 wRVU. This discrepancy in productivity may dissuade aspiring structural heart imagers from pursuing this career path.

As a result, different health systems may consider alternative payment models to make up for this discrepancy in productivity as it relates to time spent. One model may be to consider using a negotiated wRVU designation that the health system and the provider agree to. Another option may be to develop a salary-based model as opposed to productivity-based model.[53] This is an area of interest among specialty societies and advocacy is ongoing.

SUMMARY

Technological advancements in SHD procedures have mirrored those in interventional imaging capabilities. Our capacity to reliably image complex cardiac structures has improved with the advent of more reliable and efficient transducers of superior imaging quality paired with software and hardware advances allowing real-time, large volume image manipulation specific to the procedure being performed. Advanced imaging programs have evolved to train interventional imagers although with variation in focus, some more MDCT and CMR while others echocardiography focused. Training imagers to guide procedures require the development of a 3D perspective that easily moves between modalities. The value of an interventional imager is not only in the procedure room but also in the pre-procedural assessment, procedure planning, and post-procedure assessment. They must have the unique perspective to understand anatomic nuances across all imaging modalities and recommend the one suited for the specified pathology or procedure.

Training should start in general fellowship with early learning of processing 3D volumes. This skill is imperative for imagers, structural, and coronary interventionalists who are often able to "see" 3D images on a 2D fluoroscopy screen. Manipulation of 3D MDCT volumes to answer specific structural questions is the gateway to developing a perspective that spans other modalities. In general fellowship, a strong focus on MDCT is imperative regardless of future practice plans. In post-fellowship imaging training, MDCT must be taught with echocardiography. Finally, in programs that focus on MDCT and CMR, TEE should also be highlighted to allow the trainee to seamlessly move through the modalities.

As technology advances, imaging tools and software continue to evolve to allow more consistent images with less effort. This allows us as a group to be better at performing today's procedures. Success with tomorrow's procedures will require interventional imagers with a developed flexible and creative perspective allowing them to easily meld modalities with patient anatomies and their unique procedures.

DISCLOSURE

The authors have nothing to disclose.

REFERENCES

1. Wu C, Vasseur B, Maisel W. The march of transcatheter aortic valve replacement therapy—US Food and Drug administration perspectives on device approval for patients at low surgical risk. JAMA Cardiology 2020;5(1):5–6.

2. Carroll JD, Mack MJ, Vemulapalli S, et al. STS-ACC TVT registry of transcatheter aortic valve replacement. J Am Coll Cardiol 2020;76(21):2492–516.

3. Grover FL, Vemulapalli S, Carroll JD, et al. 2016 annual report of the society of thoracic surgeons/ American college of cardiology transcatheter valve therapy registry. J Am Coll Cardiol 2017;69(10): 1215–30.

4. Davidson LJ, Davidson CJ. Transcatheter treatment of valvular heart disease: a review. JAMA 2021; 325(24):2480–94.

5. Sorajja P, Whisenant B, Hamid N, et al. Transcatheter repair for patients with tricuspid regurgitation. N Engl J Med 2023;388(20):1833–42.

6. Lurz P, Stephan von Bardeleben R, Weber M, et al. Transcatheter edge-to-edge repair for treatment of tricuspid regurgitation. J Am Coll Cardiol 2021; 77(3):229–39.

7. Nickenig G, Weber M, Lurz P, et al. Transcatheter edge-to-edge repair for reduction of tricuspid regurgitation: 6-month outcomes of the TRILUMINATE single-arm study. Lancet 2019;394(10213): 2002–11.

8. Holzer RJ, Hijazi ZM. Transcatheter pulmonary valve replacement: State of the art. Cathet Cardiovasc Interv 2016;87(1):117–28.

9. O'Byrne ML, Glatz AC, Mercer-Rosa L, et al. Trends in pulmonary valve replacement in children and adults with tetralogy of fallot. Am J Cardiol 2015; 115(1):118–24.

10. Bulut MO, Yucel IK, Kucuk M, et al. Initial Experience with the Nit-Occlud ASD-R: Short-Term Results. Pediatr Cardiol 2016;37(7):1258–65.

11. Pedra CAC, Pedra SF, Costa RN, et al. Mid-term outcomes after percutaneous closure of the secundum atrial septal defect with the figulla-occlutech device. J Intervent Cardiol 2016;29(2):208–15.

12. Stout KK, Daniels CJ, Aboulhosn JA, et al. 2018 AHA/ACC Guideline for the Management of Adults With Congenital Heart Disease. J Am Coll Cardiol 2019;73(12):e81–192.

13. Roberson DA, Cui W, Patel D, et al. Three-dimensional transesophageal echocardiography of atrial septal defect: a qualitative and quantitative anatomic study. J Am Soc Echocardiogr 2011; 24(6):600–10.

14. Faletra F, Scarpini S, Moreo A, et al. Color Doppler echocardiographic assessment of atrial septal defect size: correlation with surgical measurements. J Am Soc Echocardiogr 1991;4(5):429–34.

15. Kanderian AS, Gillinov AM, Pettersson GB, et al. Success of surgical left atrial appendage closure: assessment by transesophageal echocardiography. J Am Coll Cardiol 2008;52(11):924–9.

16. Nishimura M, Lupercio-Lopez F, Hsu JC. Left atrial appendage electrical isolation as a target in atrial fibrillation. JACC Clin Electrophysiol 2019;5(4): 407–16.

17. Asmarats L, Rodés-Cabau J. Percutaneous left atrial appendage closure: current devices and clinical outcomes. Circulation: cardiovascular interventions 2017;10(11):e005359.

18. Pacha HM, Al-Khadra Y, Soud M, et al. Percutaneous devices for left atrial appendage occlusion: a contemporary review. World J Cardiol 2019; 11(2):57.

19. Suradi H, Hijazi Z. Left atrial appendage closure: outcomes and challenges. Neth Heart J 2017;25: 143–51.

20. Osmancik P, Herman D, Neuzil P, et al. Left atrial appendage closure versus direct oral anticoagulants in high-risk patients with atrial fibrillation. J Am Coll Cardiol 2020;75(25):3122–35.

21. Lindeboom JJ, Coylewright M, Etnel JR, et al. Shared decision making in the heart team: current team attitudes and review. Structural Heart 2021; 5(2):163–7.

22. Cartlidge TR, Bing R, Kwiecinski J, et al. Contrast-enhanced computed tomography assessment of aortic stenosis. Heart 2021;107(23):1905–11.

23. Otto CM, Kumbhani DJ, Alexander KP, et al. 2017 ACC expert consensus decision pathway for transcatheter aortic valve replacement in the management of adults with aortic stenosis: a report of the American College of Cardiology Task Force on Clinical Expert Consensus Documents. J Am Coll Cardiol 2017;69(10):1313–46.

24. Baumgartner HC, Hung JC-C, Bermejo J, et al. Recommendations on the echocardiographic assessment of aortic valve stenosis: a focused update from the European Association of Cardiovascular Imaging and the American Society of Echocardiography. Eur Heart J Cardiovasc Imaging 2017;18(3): 254–75.

25. Abramowitz Y, Maeno Y, Chakravarty T, et al. Aortic angulation attenuates procedural success following self-expandable but not balloon-expandable TAVR. JACC (J Am Coll Cardiol): Cardiovascular Imaging 2016;9(8):964–72.

26. Salgado RA, Leipsic JA, Shivalkar B, et al. Preprocedural CT evaluation of transcatheter aortic valve replacement: what the radiologist needs to know. Radiographics 2014;34(6):1491–514.

27. Wiegerinck EM, Van Kesteren F, Van Mourik MS, et al. An up-to-date overview of the most recent transcatheter implantable aortic valve prostheses. Expet Rev Med Dev 2016;13(1):31–45.
28. Tanis W, Suchá D, Laufer W, et al. Multidetector-row computed tomography for prosthetic heart valve dysfunction: is concomitant non-invasive coronary angiography possible before redo-surgery? Eur Radiol 2015;25:1623–30.
29. Blanke P, Soon J, Dvir D, et al. Computed tomography assessment for transcatheter aortic valve in valve implantation: the Vancouver approach to predict anatomical risk for coronary obstruction and other considerations. Journal of Cardiovascular Computed Tomography 2016;10(6):491–9.
30. Khan JM, Greenbaum AB, Babaliaros VC, et al. The BASILICA trial: prospective multicenter investigation of intentional leaflet laceration to prevent TAVR coronary obstruction. JACC Cardiovasc Interv 2019;12(13):1240–52.
31. Tang GHL, Lerakis S, Kini A, et al. 4-dimensional transesophageal echocardiographic guidance during TAVR With BASILICA. JACC (J Am Coll Cardiol): Cardiovascular Imaging 2020;13(7):1601–14.
32. Dangas G, Nicolas J. Anticoagulation and subclinical valve thrombosis after TAVR. Washington DC: American College of Cardiology Foundation; 2022. p. 1805–7.
33. Del Trigo M, Muñoz-Garcia AJ, Wijeysundera HC, et al. Incidence, timing, and predictors of valve hemodynamic deterioration after transcatheter aortic valve replacement: multicenter registry. J Am Coll Cardiol 2016;67(6):644–55.
34. Di Biase L, Santangeli P, Anselmino M, et al. Does the left atrial appendage morphology correlate with the risk of stroke in patients with atrial fibrillation?: results from a multicenter study. J Am Coll Cardiol 2012;60(6):531–8.
35. Glikson M, Wolff R, Hindricks G, et al. EHRA/EAPCI expert consensus statement on catheter-based left atrial appendage occlusion - an update. EuroIntervention 2020;15(13):1133–80.
36. Romero J, Husain SA, Kelesidis I, et al. Detection of left atrial appendage thrombus by cardiac computed tomography in patients with atrial fibrillation. Circulation: Cardiovascular Imaging 2013;6(2):185–94.
37. Patel AR, Fatemi O, Norton PT, et al. Cardiac cycle–dependent left atrial dynamics: Implications for catheter ablation of atrial fibrillation. Heart Rhythm 2008;5(6):787–93.
38. Saw J, Fahmy P, Spencer R, et al. Comparing measurements of CT angiography, TEE, and fluoroscopy of the left atrial appendage for percutaneous closure. J Cardiovasc Electrophysiol 2016;27(4):414–22.
39. Wang DD, Eng M, Kupsky D, et al. Application of 3-dimensional computed tomographic image guidance to watchman implantation and impact on early operator learning curve: single-center experience. JACC Cardiovasc Interv 2016;9(22):2329–40.
40. Rajwani A, Nelson AJ, Shirazi MG, et al. CT sizing for left atrial appendage closure is associated with favourable outcomes for procedural safety. European Heart Journal - Cardiovascular Imaging 2016;18(12):1361–8.
41. Goitein O, Fink N, Hay I, et al. Cardiac CT Angiography (CCTA) predicts left atrial appendage occluder device size and procedure outcome. Int J Cardiovasc Imag 2017;33(5):739–47.
42. Saw J, Fahmy P, DeJong P, et al. Cardiac CT angiography for device surveillance after endovascular left atrial appendage closure. European Heart Journal - Cardiovascular Imaging 2015;16(11):1198–206.
43. Dukkipati SR, Kar S, Holmes DR, et al. Device-Related Thrombus After Left Atrial Appendage Closure. Circulation 2018;138(9):874–85.
44. *ACC 2015 Core Cardiovascular Training Statement (COCATS 4) (Revision of COCATS 3): A Report of the ACC Competency Management Committee.* J Am Coll Cardiol 2015;13.
45. Little SH, et al. Recommendations for special competency in echocardiographic guidance of structural heart disease interventions: from the American society of echocardiography. J Am Soc Echocardiogr 2023;36(4):350–65.
46. Leipsic J, et al. Core competencies in cardiac CT for imaging structural heart disease interventions. J Am Coll Cardiol Img 2019;12(12):2555–9.
47. Choi AD, et al. 2020 SCCT guideline for training cardiology and radiology trainees as independent practitioners (Level II) and advanced practitioners (Level III) in cardiovascular computed tomography: a statement from the society of cardiovascular computed tomography. Radiol Cardiothorac Imaging 2020;3(1):e200480.
48. Madan N, et al. Contemporary cardiovascular computed tomography (CCT) training: Serial surveys of the international CCT community by the fellow and resident leaders of the society of cardiovascular computed tomography (SCCT) Committee (FiRST) and SCCT future leaders program (FLP). J Cardiovasc Comput Tomogr 2023;17(3):226–30.
49. Janus SE, Karnib M, Al-Kindi SG. Reimagining training in cardiac CT for cardiology fellows. J Am Coll Cardiol 2022;79(25):2543–7.
50. Faza N, et al. Imaging in structural heart disease: the evolution of a new subspecialty. J Am Coll Cardiol Case Reports 2019;1:440–5.
51. Centers for Medicare and Medicaid. 2023. Search The Physician Fee Schedule. Available at: https://www.

cms.gov/medicare/physician-fee-schedule/search. Accessed July 17, 2023.

52. Reibolt, M. RVUs – Recent History and Background of Units of Measurement. American Association for Physician Leadership. Available at: https://www.physician leaders.org/articles/rvus-recent-history-background-units-measurement. Accessed July 17, 2023.

53. Wang D, et al. Navigating a career in structural heart disease interventional imaging. J Am Coll Cardiol Img 2018;11(12):1928–30.

54. Wang, et al. Interventional imaging for structural heart disease: challenges and new frontiers of an emerging multi-disciplinary field. Structural Heart 2019;(3):187–200.

Intracardiac Echocardiographic Guidance for Structural Heart Procedures

Current Utility as Compared to Transesophageal Echocardiography

Carter W. English, MD, Jason H. Rogers, MD,
Thomas W. Smith, MD*

KEYWORDS

- Structural heart disease • Intracardiac echocardiography • Transesophageal echocardiography

---

KEY POINTS

- Intracardiac echocardiography (ICE) can provide many advantages when transesophageal echocardiographic (TEE) imaging is limited or contraindicated during structural heart procedures.
- With the development of volume 3-dimensional ICE and multiplanar reconstruction (MPR), an imaging specialist can reproduce a structural assessment similar to 3-dimensional TEE and MPR acquisition with a favorable safety profile.
- No universal standards have been established on how to perform ICE-guided imaging for various structural heart procedures, advising a need for education on how to confidently perform ICE intraoperatively.

 Video content accompanies this article at http://www.interventional.theclinics.com.

INTRODUCTION

Over the past decade, technological advancements in the image processing and clarity of cardiac ultrasound have provided new avenues for effective visualization of cardiac structures during interventionalist and electrophysiologist procedures. Intracardiac echocardiography (ICE) has been increasingly adopted with limited procedural risk when used for imaging guidance during a procedure.[1] With the development of volume 3-dimensional ICE and transesophageal echocardiographic (TEE) imaging with application of multiplanar reconstruction (MPR)

programs, a precise intraoperative assessment can provide real-time guidance even with complex anatomy with suboptimal views. With the development of transvenous and transaortic procedures for patients at increased operative risk, ICE and TEE allow physicians to diagnose and treat complex disease states with many available imaging windows.[2] As temporal and spatial resolutions continue to improve over time, there has been a growing discussion between when to utilize ICE versus TEE. Currently, TEE remains standard for a large majority of medical institutions, although the clinical application of when to decide between TEE and ICE

Division of Cardiovascular Medicine, Department of Internal Medicine, University of California – Davis Medical Center, 4860 Y Street, Suite 2820, Sacramento, CA 95817, USA
* Corresponding author.
E-mail address: twrsmith@ucdavis.edu

Intervent Cardiol Clin 13 (2024) 39–49
https://doi.org/10.1016/j.iccl.2023.08.008
2211-7458/24/© 2023 Elsevier Inc. All rights reserved.

should be considered. This article discusses the utilization of ICE versus TEE for various interventional procedures.

DISCUSSION

Technological Intracardiac Echocardiography and Transesophageal Echocardiographic Applications and Limitations

The technologies and equipment needed for ICE and TEE are similar, but understanding the differences can provide an intuitive analysis in understanding the practicality of using each during structural interventions. The major format for 2-dimensional ICE uses a phased-array 64-element piezoelectric crystal transducer mounted at the distal end of a steerable catheter.[3] Various 2-dimensioanl catheters are now available from different medical device companies, including Siemens, Malvern, PA (ACUSON AcuNav 4D Volume ICE catheter), Biosense Webster, Irvine, CA (NuVision), and Phillips, San Diego, CA (VeriSight Pro). Because of the variation in arrays by different manufactures, there can be specific geometric limitations for every device. For example, the Phillips Verisight Pro ICE catheter has resolution optimal at both −45° and + 45° with progressive worsening spatial resolution when approaching −90° and + 90°. The small catheter size that is used through femoral venous access has allowed ICE to guide structural procedures without general anesthesia for airway protection for intraoperative TEE. Although manufacture dependent, the frequency can range between 4 and 10 MHz and approximately 90 cm working length with an articulated segment that can be manipulated to move the catheter tip anterior/posterior and/or left/right in addition the rotational clockwise/counterclockwise. With advancement of matrix phase arrays in the past 5 years, an imaging specialist now can view an area of interest with a 90° × 90° volume acquisition, providing a comprehensive live 3-dimensional assessment of the structural anatomy of the heart. Additionally, the development of on-cart multiplanar reconstruction (MPR) gives an anatomically correct interpretation of the heart similar but not equal to TEE imaging quality. Full-color Doppler is available with ICE, although the temporal resolution is drastically reduced when 3-dimensional or MPR is applied and is lower quality compared with the TEE counterpart.

The catheter of the ICE probe is commonly placed via the common femoral vein and then guided to the right atrium to acquire a standardized first view, called home view, which directs the probe to visualize the right atrium and ventricle at 0°. From home view, the probe is manipulated by the proceduralist using anatomic landmarks to optimize the region of interest, which may include advancing the catheter trans-septal during left-side structural interventions. Although access of an ICE catheter is commonly standardized to the common femoral vein, a transjugular approach is possible for complex or suboptimal venous anatomy and often commonly used for transjugular intrahepatic portosystemic shut creations by interventional radiologists.[4] Unfortunately, at this time, the reimbursement of using ICE during structural cardiac interventions has not been established, leading to financial costs and inability to appropriately reimburse the time and effort of the proceduralist and imager during an ICE-only imaging case. This cost may be offset to some degree, as full anesthesia support may not be needed if the procedure is performed under conscious sedation.

TEE imaging has been using matrix phase-arrayed piezoelectric crystal for the past decade with the ability to acquire numerous 3-dimensional data sets to generate multiplanar reconstructions, which are of better temporal and spatial resolution compared with ICE. A standard 3-dimensional applicable TEE probe can be manipulated to an optimal field of view either within the esophagus or the fundus of the stomach by anteflexion/retroflexion, left/right, clockwise/counterclockwise movements. The location of the esophagus determines the reproducibility of standard images that can be acquired in different patients. A more lateral esophagus or decreased esophageal lumen can lead to substandard images, which may limit a proceduralist's capacity to comprehensively and safely guide a transcatheter intervention. With reproducible images, TEE can provide accurate imaging guidance and consistent results, leading to improved outcomes. Because of the anatomic constraints of intracardiac imaging, 2-dimensional ICE cannot easily view certain standard imaging planes. With the development of ICE 3-dimensional and MPR, an imaging specialist can reproduce a structural assessment similar to TEE 3-dimensional and MPR acquisitions while maintaining a similar safety profile during the procedure. Additionally, intraprocedural risk of gastrointestinal (GI) bleeding from TEE after a structural cardiac intervention is uncommon but has been reported in approximately 3% of patients. The individuals at highest risk are the elderly, those who take anticoagulants or antiplatelet therapies, and those who require longer acquisition times, causing thermal injury or high contact pressure on the esophageal mucosa leading to direct tissue trauma.[5] Unless in a unique situation, TEE-guided transcatheter procedures require anesthesia due to airway protection with the patient laying supine. Thus, the use of TEE can have increased total procedural time because of the additive time of induction, intubation, extubation, and recovery. The use of an intracardiac catheter can also result in complications including the possibility of direct heart damage/perforation, pericardial effusion/tamponade, and vascular access-related injury.

Left Atrial Appendage Occlusion

Left atrial appendage occlusion (LAAO) devices are now an established therapy to optimize patients with atrial fibrillation and prior GI or neurologic bleeding.[6,7] To ensure safe and effective device deployment, careful planning is performed prior to procedure using imaging modalities such as electrocardiogram (ECG)-gated cardiac computed tomography (CT) angiography or TEE to acquire accurate appendage landing orifice measurements for sizing of the LAAC device. TEE remains the main imaging modality in conjunction with fluoroscopy to guide LAAO device delivery. Precise atrial septal access for trans-septal puncture positioning is paramount to avoid adverse outcomes including off-axis device deployment or peridevice leak. The typical trans-septal puncture location is in the inferior-posterior quadrant of the fossa ovalis[8] (Video 1), although other trans-septal crossing locations may be required for certain LAA anatomies. After guidance of the sheath through the atrial septum and into the left atrium (LA), real-time imaging guidance allows the proceduralist to reconfirm appropriate LAA orifice sizing prior to device engagement into the appendage (Fig. 1, see Video 1). Furthermore, imaging is used to guide the device safely into the appendage and observe it deploy in real time to ensure no dislodgment or perforation occurs. After deployment, echocardiography provides assessment of device seal, position, and presence of any perivalvular leaks. If positioning is suboptimal, the device is captured, repositioned, and redeployed prior to confirming no leak and release of the device. Follow-up imaging is typically performed with TEE, although many sites are utilizing cardiac CT to assess closure and positioning.

The Society of Cardiovascular Angiography and Interventions and the Heart Rhythm Society have strongly recommended that either TEE or ICE is utilized for LAAO intraprocedural guidance.[8] For ICE, the probe is generally inserted through the trans-septal puncture and into the LA to provide optimal procedural guidance as right atrium (RA) position leads to decreased resolution and thus variable measurement parameters for LAAO device sizing. Some operators have placed the ICE catheter into the coronary sinus or pulmonary artery to image the LAA. While in the LA, the ICE probe must be manipulated to acquire images that are comparable to TEE standards for LAAO guidance. These views are commonly achieved by retroflexion within the LA, insertion into the left upper pulmonary vein, and positioning above the mitral annulus.

To decide the utility between TEE and ICE imaging for intraprocedural guidance, the LAAO Italian Multicenter Registry acquired data from 604 LAAC Amplatzer device procedures at 16 separate medical centers in Italy and compared 417 TEE-guided with 187 ICE-guided LAAO procedures. There were no significant differences in procedural success, total complication rates, or cerebral ischemic event rates.[9] Of note, CT was the predominant modality used for preprocedural assessment, and there was about a 16-minute increase in procedural time using an ICE-guided approach. Pre-CT assessment did not affect intraprocedural complications.[9] When performing an LAAC procedure using a Watchman device, similar outcomes and complications data were seen between TEE-guided and ICE-guided patients in a multicenter study performed in the United States.[10]

A growing amount of evidence demonstrates ICE-guided workflows are comparable to TEE-guided workflows during a left atrial appendage occlusion device procedure. A metanalysis of 9 separate studies (retrospective) comparing the outcomes of 2-dimensional ICE versus TEE from 2017 to 2020 for LAAC devices in patients with atrial fibrillation with high bleeding risk determined comparable procedural success, procedural duration, periprocedural complications, fluoroscopy time, and contrast volume between both imaging modalities with limited publication bias observed.[11] The length of stay for ICE-guided procedures was lower than for TEE. Data with volume 3-dimensional ICE remain an emerging topic that may allow for better results compared with TEE. A prospective, multicenter study (ICE LAA Study) recently and strongly suggested ICE is an effective tool for guidance of Watchman FLX devices without conversion to TEE and with 0% significant peridevice leak of greater than 5 mm. An ICE LAA study further provided evidence that ICE for Watchman is safe and cost-effective.[12] ICE

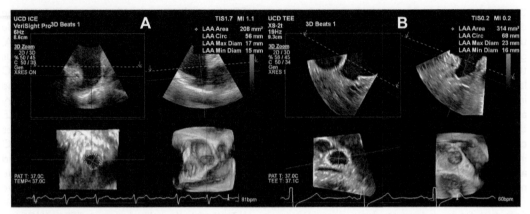

Fig. 1. Multiplanar reconstruction using ICE-guidance (A) and TEE-guidance (B) to optimize measurement of the left atrial appendage orifice sizing in a similar fashion to how multiplanar reconstruction via CT estimates orifice size to guide device sizing for a patient. In the left upper orthogonal view, the cross-section plane is guided by the position of left circumflex artery.

compared with TEE was comparable to safety, cost, and feasibility, although the downstream costs of not requiring general anesthesia and postprocedural turnaround may suggest a financial benefit toward the application of ICE versus TEE for LAAC devices.

Although preference remains regarding TEE-guided versus ICE guided imaging for LAAC, further 3-dimensional MPR software additions to ICE have provided a new avenue of procedural accuracy that may further place ICE as a preferable modality, especially with individuals with prior resolved GI bleeding. Furthermore, the use of MPR is reproducible and can be standardized using a similar method to preprocedural CT, setting a comparable standard for preprocedural, intraprocedural, and postprocedural imaging for LAAC devices (see Fig. 1; Fig. 2, Videos 2–4).

Patent Foramen Ovale/Atrial Septal Defect Closure

A congenital/iatrogenic atrial septal defect (ASD) and a large patent foramen ovale (PFO) can inflict long-term complications of arrhythmias, right heart failure, and paradoxic embolic stroke which often arise in adulthood.[13] Transcatheter closure of ASD and PFO defects is a viable option for patients who want to avoid surgery. The use of ICE in addition to TEE for ASD and PFO closures has been documented in pediatric interventions for over 2 decades.[14] Although ICE is ideal for intraprocedural image guidance, the authors still recommend preprocedural high-quality TEE imaging for any ASD or complex PFO to confirm the size and presence of the defect. During the closure procedure, the ICE catheter is commonly

inserted after venous access is achieved (Fig. 3). ICE guidance can allow for a larger variety of angles to visualize and interpret the atrial septum and its defect, particularly improving visualization of the inferior rim compared with TEE guidance.[15,16] (Fig. 4). The ICE probe can be positioned in the upper and middle RA with posterior and rightward flexion to acquire the inferior and superior rims of an ASD and to acquire an ICE bicaval view.[17] The ICE catheter can be manipulated to tilt leftward to obtain a septal short-axis and appreciate the posterior and anterior rims of an ASD. ICE probe home view should be used to sweep the area of interest to ensure no sinus venosus-ASD is present.[17] Once an ASD/PFO is appropriately visualized, measurements of the defect should be acquired around the rims.[17] A sizing balloon may be deployed across an ASD under ICE to appreciate any color-Doppler flow with the diameter of the balloon measured in multiple imaging plane.[17] Once ready to deploy a septal occluding device, the ICE probe is positioned in the septal long axis view (posterior and rightward flexion) to observe the steps of device closure and ensure the device is away from pulmonary veins and the LA appendage when engaged in the left atrium.[17] (Fig. 5). After the procedure, the ASD closure device is evaluated for any closure leaks.

ICE guidance assists in seeing visual details of the atrial septum more clearly, with the advantage of limiting any need for anesthesia while the patient remains supine during the procedure.[18] Long-term follow-up after ICE-guided ASD closure has been observed with excellent rates of procedural success and avoidance of incorrect device sizing and selection.[19] Comparative analysis of

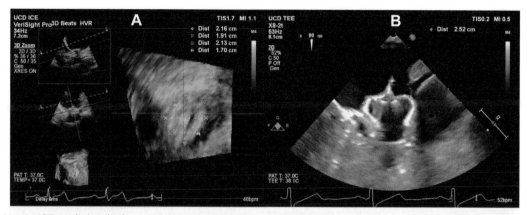

Fig. 2. ICE-guided multiplanar reconstruction with orthogonal views (A) positioned to align a deployed LAAC device into the left atrial appendage. Under MPR, multiple measures can be performed to assess the amount of device compression after development. TEE-guided measurement (B) of LAAC device at the superior and inferior border to assess device compression after deployment.

ICE versus TEE from 2003 to 2014 demonstrated a fivefold increase in ICE guidance in the closure of interatrial communications, with similar outcomes, complications, cost, and shorter length of stay.[20] Additionally, a large meta-analysis recently performed involving 11 studies including 4748 individuals (2386 ICE-guided, 2362 TEE-guided) that compared the procedural outcomes of PFO and ASD closures demonstrated a significant decrease in fluoroscopy time, procedural time, length of hospital stay, and adverse events, including arrhythmias and vascular complications in the ICE-guided group. No difference in closure outcomes were seen.[21]

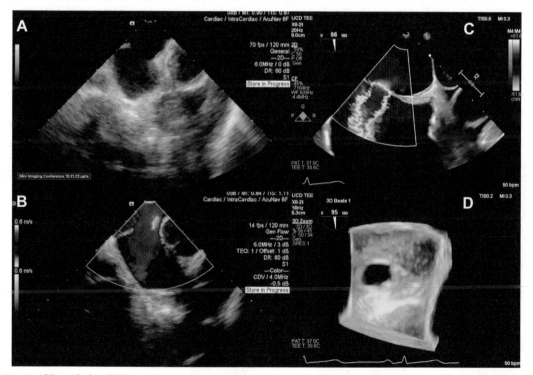

Fig. 3. ICE-guided and TEE-guided atrial septal defect with visualization of the septal defect. (A) 2-dimensional ICE imaging of an anterior superior septum secundum atrial septal defect with color-Doppler (B) predominant left-to-right shunt. (C) 2-dimensional TEE imaging of a midlocated septum secundum atrial septal defect with color-Doppler demonstrating left-to-right shunt and (D) 3-dimensional volumetric reconstruction.

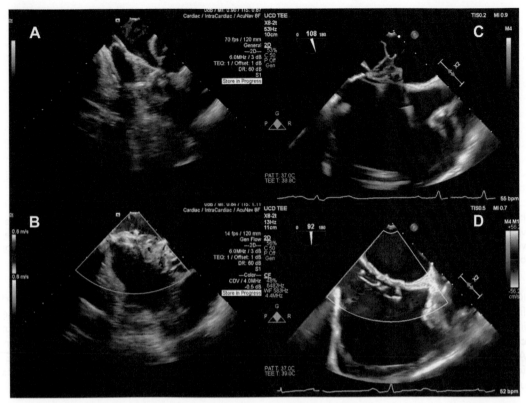

Fig. 4. ICE-guided (A, B) and TEE-guided (C, D) imaging of atrial septal defect closure via Gore Cardioform device with deployment of left atrial side (A, C) and completion of ASD closure and assessment via color-Doppler (B, D).

Mitral Valve Transcatheter Edge-to-Edge Repair

With recent guidelines and randomized control trials demonstrating the utility of transcatheter mitral valve edge-to-edge repair (M-TEER), 3-dimensional echocardiographic imaging is paramount for appropriate trans-septal puncture at an appropriate height from the mitral annulus, ensuring device capture of the anterior and posterior leaflets, and evaluating severity of mitral regurgitation and reduction after deployment of the device.[22] TEE has been the primary mode

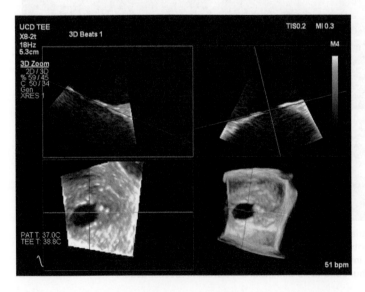

Fig. 5. TEE-guided MPR of a midoriented septum secundum atrial septal defect.

of imaging in M-TEER procedures with the benefit of being able to visualize multiple planes in real time during deployment of an M-TEER device. With the advent of improved imaging, ICE has been proposed as an alternative method to guide M-TEER procedures (Video 5). The first documented case of ICE-guided M-TEER was performed in 2017 on a patient who had severe mitral regurgitation but was prohibited from TEE because of a significant esophageal stricture.[23] During an M-TEER procedure, the ICE probe is advanced into the RA, where it is initially used to guide trans-septal puncture. After septal puncture is achieved, the ICE probe is advanced into the LA followed by the steerable guide catheter and M-TEER device system. Once in appropriate position within the LA, the ICE catheter can utilize multiple viewing planes in real time to approximate the TTE-equivalent of a bicommissural and "grasping" view through rightward and posterior flexion of the catheter (Video 6, Fig. 6). Furthermore, the development of ICE-based MPR provides improved accuracy in M-TEER alignment, orientation, and positioning compared with 2-dimensional imaging.[24,25] There remains difficulty in capturing the entire mitral annulus in a single view because of the closer proximity from the probe to the region of interest. Although no large retrospective observational studies are available to compare outcomes and complications using ICE-guided imaging with TEE-guided imaging, case studies have been published noting that ICE can provide unobstructed views of the intracardiac device that may in some cases be better compared with TEE imaging, although image acquisition is highly dependent on the catheter position and steerability with a smaller field of view.[26,27] Like other procedures, volume 3-dimensional ICE temporal and spatial resolution is inferior to TEE, although TEE is limited by probe positioning within the esophageal tract and downfield intracardiac device acoustic shadowing.

Transcatheter Triscuspid Valve Edge-to-Edge Repair

Severe symptomatic tricuspid regurgitation (TR) can be considered for treatment via percutaneous tricuspid TEER (T-TEER) with improvement in TR severity and quality of life.[28,29] Like M-TEER, ICE is considered an alternative approach to procedural imaging when TEE is unavailable. ICE guidance during a T-TEER procedure can overcome a significant amount of acoustic shadowing made from nearby calcified structures, thickened atrial septum, and/or device-related shadowing (prosthetic valves, pacing leads) (Video 7). Given the limitations of TEE for tricuspid valve compared with mitral valve visualization, ICE can provide adjunct views to enhance the treatment outcomes of T-TEER. Through a recent ex-vivo laboratory investigation, 3-dimensional MPR ICE was assessed for T-TEER with the observed strength of improved leaflet visualization when grasped by a device when TEE imaging is suboptimal. When viewing the tricuspid valve during T-TEER, 2-dimensional ICE demonstrates a high spatial and temporal resolution that is comparable to 2-dimensional TEE imaging.[30] Alternatively with current imaging technology, 3-dimensional MPR TEE has remarkably higher temporal and spatial resolution compared with 3-dimensional MPR ICE during T-TEER procedures (Fig. 7). A small recent case series demonstrated ICE-augmented T-TEER with standard TEE-guidance had significant reduction of TR when TEE imaging was considered suboptimal for treatment.[31,32] Because of the variable commissural standard of the tricuspid valve, orientation of the TEER depends on 3-dimensional MPR to ensure perfect alignment of the leaflets to the device to

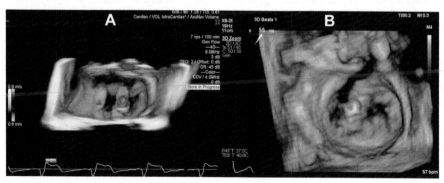

Fig. 6. ICE-guided (*A*) and TEE-guided (*B*) m-TEER with real-time 3-dimensional reconstruction with color-flow Doppler to confirmed device orientation in relationship to P2 flail for each case.

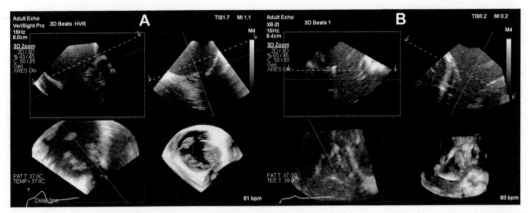

Fig. 7. ICE-guided (*A*) and TEE-guided (*B*) t-TEER procedure for 2 separate patients demonstrating utility of MPR to guide approach of treatment in real time. (*A*) ICE-directed MPR attempting optimal orientation and direction of the first anterior-septal device implantation. Orthogonal views either directed at the A-S commissure (*upper left*) or the anterior and septal leaflets (*upper right*). 3-dimensional reconstruction oriented in standard view with aortic valve positioned at 5-o'clock.

ensure no off-angled grasping that may lead to increased postprocedural TR or single-leaflet detachment[33] (Videos 8 and 9). As T-TEER continues to advance over the next decade, the utilization of ICE and TEE may provide benefit for patient outcomes given the large structural variability between patients with severe TR.

Transcatheter Aortic Valve Replacement

With the advent of cardiac valve replacement through percutaneous intervention, ICE has been proposed as an imaging modality when alternative methods are of low quality, are contraindicated, or do not address a specific need during a procedure. Transaortic valve replacement (TAVR) has been established as a safe alternative to surgical aortic valve replacement for patients with symptomatic severe aortic stenosis and either requires TEE or TTE imaging guidance in conjunction with measurements obtained from pre-procedural ECG-gate CT.[34] Current workflows utilize TTE for monitoring, with guidance primarily done with fluoroscopy. In the rare instances where CT scans are contraindicated, TEE may be utilized to assess annular and coronary anatomy. In the rare instance where TEE is contraindicated and real-time imaging is necessary, ICE is a tertiary alternative for procedural guidance (Video 10). If used, an ICE catheter is entered through standard femoral venous access with advancement of the probe to the superior cavo-atrial junction and can visualize the ascending aorta, transcatheter heart valve, and annulus to confirm appropriate alignment and deployment.[35] After deployment, the ICE catheter can be withdrawn into the RA

with the short axis of the transcatheter heart valve being visualized by guiding the probe to tilt anterior and at approximately 90° where paravalvular leak can be accurately assessed.[35,36] In cases when treatment is needed following TAVR, such as with a perivalvular leak, ICE can guide the interventionalist (see Video 10). To assess adjacent structures, the ICE catheter may be directed into the right ventricle and directed at the ventricular septum to assess the mitral valve, left ventricular outflow tract, and left ventricular cavity.[35]

Transcatheter Mitral Valve Replacement

Transcatheter mitral valve replacement (TMVR) devices have recently been utilized for severe mitral regurgitation or mitral stenosis. Various case studies have witnessed the application of ICE during TMVR procedures where the ICE catheter is manipulated in the same fashion as during an M-TEER procedure with the ability to gain transeptal access, imaging prior to TMVR device deployment, and post-deployment assessment for device or paravalvular leak.[37,38] ICE has been proposed as a safe and effective method for TMVR in valve-in-ring, valve-in-valve, or valve-in-MAC patients.[39] Given the novel application of transcatheter tricuspid valve replacement, minimal ICE-guided applications have been documented, including ICE guiding a SAPIEN 3 valve within a Mosaic bioprosthetic surgical valve after severe regurgitation was observed.[40] When imaging limitations from advanced kidney disease, severe pulmonary hypertension, or recurrent GI bleeding make general anesthesia and TEE unapproachable,

Table 1
Intracardiac echocardiography for structural heart interventions

Pros	Cons
No transesophageal echocardiography required	Limited vendor options
Conscious sedation	Unclear procedural reimbursement
Improved scheduling workflow for operative time	May require additional operator during procedure
Patient comfort	Physicians lack of expertise and familiarity with use
Decreased bleeding risk	Increased intracardiac injury risk
Independent of esophageal position	Higher learning curve to acquire appropriate image
Decreased probe manipulation during procedure	Unable to reuse/recycle probe
Superior imaging for right-sided interventions	Limited (although developing) clinical evidence

careful use of ICE guidance during a procedure under experienced hands may give the interventionalist the opportunity to provide care to individuals who have limited options.

SUMMARY

ICE-guided imaging has been described for various common or innovative procedures. As technological advances continue to improve the spatial and temporal resolution, 3-dimensional reconstructions, and artifactual-correction of echocardiography, structural cases will acquire improved precision to patient's specific conditions and comorbidities. TEE remains a paramount imaging modality commonly used and taught throughout structural imaging. When TEE only provides limited data or is contraindicated, ICE should be considered an alternative supplement to any structural procedure if care is taken to understand the learning curve and differences compared with TEE (Table 1). No universal standards have been established on how to perform ICE-guided imaging for various structural procedures, demonstrating the academic calling for improvement in ICE education to improve these applications beyond structural cardiac centers of excellence.

TEE probes, with ample engineering space relative to ICE catheters, will likely see imaging advancements that supersede ICE advancements over the foreseeable future. TEE probes will benefit from gradual reduction in size, improved probe manipulation, and reduced risk of esophageal injury or trauma. Nevertheless, ICE remains a beneficial tool to augment TEE-procedural images. Advances in artificial intelligence may potentially automate various steps to provide optimal imaging during complex structural

procedures and improve imaging access and consistency that is currently reliant on an experienced, dedicated structural imager. Attempts to utilize one modality over the other to reduce cost or improve operational efficiency without prioritizing the superior imaging modality for a given anatomy will result in inferior procedural results. ICE should not be viewed as a replacement for TEE, but more as a complementary imaging tool for effective patient care. Although standard in interatrial septum interventions, 2-dimensional and 3-dimensional ICE best practices are developing for a broad range of structural heart procedures. As transcatheter structural options grow, centers with expert imagers and operators can discuss before procedure which imaging modality best matches the unique characteristics of the patient and the procedure.

CLINICS CARE POINTS

- ICE, like TEE, is safe for patients requiring a structural heart intervention, including LAAO device, PFO/ASD closure, m-TEER, t-TEER, and transcatheter valve replacements.

- ICE is not a future replacement for TEE imaging for structural heart procedures, but rather a supplementary tool to further augment procedural outcomes and reduce complications.

- Advancement in echocardiogram innovation and technology provide ICE with new modes of imaging, such as live MPR, further augments pre-/intra-/postprocedural assessment, especially in nonstandard, complex cases.

DISCLOSURE

C.W. English: nothing to disclose; J.H. Rogers: consultant to Abbott, Boston Scientific, and Laminar. T.W. Smith: consultant to Abbot, Laminar, Gore Medical, and Novo Nordisk.

SUPPLEMENTARY DATA

Supplementary data related to this article can be found online at https://doi.org/10.1016/j.iccl.2023.08.008.

REFERENCES

1. Silvestry FE, Kadakia MB, Willhide J, et al. Initial experience with a novel real-time three-dimensional intracardiac ultrasound system to guide percutaneous cardiac structural interventions: a phase 1 feasibility study of volume intracardiac echocardiography in the assessment of patients with structural heart disease undergoing percutaneous transcatheter therapy. J Am Soc Echocardiogr 2014;27(9):978–83.

2. Enriquez A, Saenz LC, Rosso R, et al. Use of intracardiac echocardiography in interventional cardiology: working with the anatomy rather than fighting it. Circulation 2018;137(21):2278–94.

3. Vitulano N, Pazzano V, Pelargonio G, et al. Technology update: intracardiac echocardiography - a review of the literature. Med Devices (Auckl) 2015;8:231–9.

4. Grimsbo MC, Brown MA, Lindquist JD, et al. Intracardiac echocardiography-guided TIPS: a primer for new operators. Semin Intervent Radiol 2020;37(4):405–13.

5. Hasnie AA, Parcha V, Hawi R, et al. Complications associated with transesophageal echocardiography in transcatheter structural cardiac interventions. J Am Soc Echocardiogr 2023;36(4):381–90.

6. Reddy VY, Doshi SK, Kar S, et al. 5-year outcomes after left atrial appendage closure: from the PREVAIL and PROTECT AF trials. J Am Coll Cardiol 2017;70(24):2964–75.

7. Lakkireddy D, Thaler D, Ellis CR, et al. Amplatzer Amulet Left Atrial Appendage Occluder versus Watchman Device for stroke prophylaxis (Amulet IDE): a randomized, controlled trial. Circulation 2021;144(19):1543–52.

8. Saw J, Holmes DR, Cavalcante JL, et al. SCAI/HRS expert consensus statement on transcatheter left atrial appendage closure. Heart Rhythm 2023;20(5):e1–16.

9. Berti S, Pastormerlo LE, Santoro G, et al. Intracardiac versus transesophageal echocardiographic guidance for left atrial appendage occlusion: the LAAO Italian multicenter registry. JACC Cardiovasc Interv 2018;11(11):1086–92.

10. Alkhouli M, Chaker Z, Alqahtani F, et al. Outcomes of routine intracardiac echocardiography to guide left atrial appendage occlusion. JACC Clin Electrophysiol 2020;6(4):393–400.

11. Jhand A, Thandra A, Gwon Y, et al. Intracardiac echocardiography versus transesophageal echocardiography for left atrial appendage closure: an updated meta-analysis and systematic review. Am J Cardiovasc Dis 2020;10(5):538–47.

12. Nielsen-Kudsk JE, Berti S, Caprioglio F, et al. Intracardiac echocardiography to guide Watchman FLX implantation: the ICE LAA study. JACC Cardiovasc Interv 2023;16(6):643–51.

13. Geva T, Martins JD, Wald RM. Atrial septal defects. Lancet 2014;383(9932):1921–32.

14. Hijazi Z, Wang Z, Cao Q, et al. Transcatheter closure of atrial septal defects and patent foramen ovale under intracardiac echocardiographic guidance: feasibility and comparison with transesophageal echocardiography. Catheter Cardiovasc Interv 2001;52(2):194–9.

15. Koenig P, Cao QL. Echocardiographic guidance of transcatheter closure of atrial septal defects: is intracardiac echocardiography better than transesophageal echocardiography? Pediatr Cardiol 2005;26(2):135–9.

16. Assaidi A, Sumian M, Mauri L, et al. Transcatheter closure of complex atrial septal defects is efficient under intracardiac echocardiographic guidance. Arch Cardiovasc Dis 2014;107(12):646–53.

17. Silvestry FE, Cohen MS, Armsby LB, et al. Guidelines for the echocardiographic assessment of atrial septal defect and patent foramen ovale: from the American Society of Echocardiography and Society for Cardiac Angiography and Interventions. J Am Soc Echocardiogr 2015;28(8):910–58.

18. Bartel T, Konorza T, Arjumand J, et al. Intracardiac echocardiography is superior to conventional monitoring for guiding device closure of interatrial communications. Circulation 2003;107(6):795–7.

19. Rigatelli G, Dell'Avvocata F, Cardaioli P, et al. Five-year follow-up of transcatheter intracardiac echocardiography-assisted closure of interatrial shunts. Cardiovasc Revasc Med 2011;12(6):355–61.

20. Alqahtani F, Bhirud A, Aljohani S, et al. Intracardiac versus transesophageal echocardiography to guide transcatheter closure of interatrial communications: Nationwide trend and comparative analysis. J Interv Cardiol 2017;30(3):234–41.

21. Lan Q, Wu F, Ye X, et al. Intracardiac vs. transesophageal echocardiography for guiding transcatheter closure of interatrial communications: a systematic review and meta-analysis. Front Cardiovasc Med 2023;10:1082663.

22. Stone GW, Lindenfeld J, Abraham WT, et al. Transcatheter mitral-valve repair in patients with heart failure. N Engl J Med 2018;379(24):2307–18.

23. Patzelt J, Schreieck J, Camus E, et al. Percutaneous mitral valve edge-to-edge repair using volume intracardiac echocardiography-first in human experience. CASE (Phila) 2017;1(1):41–3.

24. Sanchez CE, Yakubov SJ, Singh G, et al. 4-dimensional intracardiac echocardiography in transcatheter mitral valve repair with the Mitraclip System. JACC Cardiovasc Imaging 2021;14(10):2033–40.

25. Yap J, Rogers JH, Aman E, et al. MitraClip implantation guided by volumetric intracardiac echocardiography: technique and feasibility in patients intolerant to transesophageal echocardiography. Cardiovasc Revasc Med 2021;28S:85–8.

26. Blusztein DI, Lehenbauer K, Sitticharoenchai P, et al. 3D intracardiac echocardiography in mitral transcatheter edge-to-edge repair: when TEE is hard to stomach. JACC Case Rep 2022;4(13):780–6.

27. Hoffman Scott J, Hari Pawan K, Sarcia PJ, Reiff Chris J, et al. Mitral valve transcatheter edge-to-edge repair performed exclusively with 3-dimensional intracardiac echocardiography and moderate sedation. J Soc Cardiovasc Angiography Interventions 2023;100537.

28. Lurz P, Stephan von Bardeleben R, Weber M, et al. Transcatheter edge-to-edge repair for treatment of tricuspid regurgitation. J Am Coll Cardiol 2021;77(3):229–39.

29. Sorajja P, Whisenant B, Hamid N, et al. Transcatheter repair for patients with tricuspid regurgitation. N Engl J Med 2023;388(20):1833–42.

30. Chadderdon SM, Eleid MF, Thaden JJ, et al. Three-dimensional intracardiac echocardiography for tricuspid transcatheter edge-to-edge repair. Struct Heart 2022;6(4):100071.

31. Curio J, Abulgasim K, Kasner M, et al. Intracardiac echocardiography to enable successful edge-to-edge transcatheter tricuspid valve repair in patients with insufficient TEE quality. Clin Hemorheol Microcirc 2020;76(2):199–210.

32. Eleid MF, Alkhouli M, Thaden JJ, et al. Utility of intracardiac echocardiography in the early experience of transcatheter edge to edge tricuspid valve repair. Circ Cardiovasc Interv 2021;14(10):e011118.

33. Hahn RT, Nabauer M, Zuber M, et al. Intraprocedural imaging of transcatheter tricuspid valve interventions. JACC Cardiovasc Imaging 2019;12(3):532–53.

34. Mack MJ, Leon MB, Thourani VH, et al. Transcatheter aortic-valve replacement with a balloon-expandable valve in low-risk patients. N Engl J Med 2019;380(18):1695–705.

35. Bartel T, Edris A, Velik-Salchner C, et al. Intracardiac echocardiography for guidance of transcatheter aortic valve implantation under monitored sedation: a solution to a dilemma? Eur Heart J Cardiovasc Imaging 2016;17(1):1–8.

36. Bykhovsky MR, Atianzar K, Agarwal S, et al. Use of intracardiac echocardiography to differentiate post-transcatheter aortic valve replacement valve insufficiency masquerading as paravalvular leak. CASE (Phila) 2020;4(3):111–4.

37. Bhardwaj B, Lantz G, Golwala H, et al. Transcatheter valve-in-valve mitral valve replacement using 4D intracardiac echocardiogram and conscious sedation. Struct Heart 2022;6(3):100046.

38. Cubeddu RJ, Sarkar A, Navas V, et al. 'Minimalist approach' for transcatheter mitral valve replacement using intracardiac echocardiography and conscious sedation: a case series. Eur Heart J Case Rep 2020;4(3):1–5.

39. Pommier T, Guenancia C, Sagnard A, et al. Safety and efficacy of transcatheter mitral valve replacement guided by intracardiac echocardiography. JACC Cardiovasc Interv 2021;14(14):1620–2.

40. Saji M, Ailawadi G, Izarnotegui V, et al. Intracardiac echocardiography during transcatheter tricuspid valve-in-valve implantation. Cardiovasc Interv Ther 2018;33(3):285–7.

Anomalous Coronary Arteries

A State-of-the-Art Approach

Silvana Molossi, MD, PhD[a,b,]*, Tam Doan, MD[a,b],
Shagun Sachdeva, MD[a,b]

KEYWORDS

- Sudden cardiac death • Anomalous aortic origin of a coronary artery • Coronary artery anomalies
- Advanced imaging • Cardiac catheterization

KEY POINTS

- Congenital anomalies of the coronary arteries may affect up to 1% of the population and lead to myocardial ischemia and sudden death.
- Echocardiography can diagnose anomalous coronaries in up to 95% of patients, though advanced imaging has greatly enhanced the ability to define morphologic features that impact outcome.
- Risk stratification remains a challenge in the setting of anomalous aortic origin of a coronary artery (AAOCA), and myocardial functional studies under provocative stress greatly contribute to management decision-making.
- Standardized approach to the evaluation and management of patients with coronary anomalies, with data gathering and collaboration among institutions, are paramount to optimize outcomes in this population.
- Optimal strategies in management will foster a safer environment for patients with coronary anomalies to engage in exercise and sports participation, essential components to successful and healthier lives.

INTRODUCTION

Congenital anomalies of the coronary arteries represent a varied group of lesions and are seen in less than 1% to 5% of the population, depending on method of diagnosis.[1,2] Embryologic development of the coronary artery is not completely understood, although altered coronary embryogenesis may result in abnormal coronary origins from the aorta or pulmonary artery or incomplete development leading to coronary fistulae or sinusoids. It can occur as an isolated anomaly or in association with other congenital heart diseases. Although many coronary artery anomalies are detected as incidental findings with little to no significant consequence, approximately 20% of all may have a potential risk of coronary ischemia leading to myocardial infarction, arrhythmia, and sudden cardiac death (SCD).[1-3] This report focuses on the anatomy, physiology, diagnostic strategy, and management of isolated anomalous origin of a coronary artery from the aorta and from the pulmonary artery.

This article originally appeared in *Cardiology Clinics*, Volume 41 Issue 1, February 2023.

[a] Coronary Artery Anomalies Program, Texas Children's Hospital, 6651 Main Street, MC E1920, Houston, TX 77030, USA; [b] The Lillie Frank Abercrombie Section of Cardiology, Texas Children's Hospital, Baylor College of Medicine, 6651 Main Street, MC E1920, Houston, TX 77030, USA

* Corresponding author. Coronary Artery Anomalies Program, Texas Children's Hospital, 6651 Main Street, MC E1920, Houston, TX 77030.

E-mail address: smolossi@bcm.edu

ANOMALOUS AORTIC ORIGIN OF A CORONARY ARTERY

Prevalence and Clinical Significance

The true prevalence of anomalous aortic origin of a coronary artery (AAOCA) in the general population remains unknown because studies have focused primarily on symptomatic patients. The estimated frequency of anomalous aortic origin of the left coronary artery (AAOLCA) is 0.03% to 0.15%, whereas that of anomalous aortic origin of the right coronary artery (AAORCA) is 0.28% to 0.92%.[1,4] AAOCA is known to be the second leading cause of SCD in young athletes, estimated to be responsible for 15% to 20% of sudden death in this population.[3,5] The risk of SCD seems highest in young individuals, particularly during or following a period of strenuous exertion, and particularly in those with interarterial and intramural AAOLCA. Studies of adult cohorts with AAORCA undergoing conservative therapy have observed a very low mortality (<1%) in about 1 to 5 years of follow-up.[4,6]

Anatomic subtypes and pathophysiology

This anomaly can involve either the right coronary originating from the left sinus of Valsalva (reportedly more common) or the left coronary originating from the right sinus of Valsalva (Fig. 1), and rarely more posteriorly from the noncoronary sinus or near the posterior commissure with or without an intramural course.[7]

Several pathophysiologic mechanisms have been postulated for the occurrence of sudden cardiac arrest (SCA)/SCD in patients with AAOCA. These include occlusion and/or compression of the anomalous coronary artery (intramural segment, interarterial course) and ostial abnormalities (slit-like and stenotic ostium), particularly during exercise, leading to myocardial ischemia and development of ventricular arrhythmia.[8] In a study by Basso and colleagues, of 27 individuals who experienced SCD due to AAOCA, only 10 presented with symptoms before the event.[5] Given the significant number of patients that are asymptomatic before a critical adverse cardiac event, this highlights difficulties in evaluating patients at risk for adverse sudden cardiac events.

Clinical evaluation

Clinical Presentation and Diagnosis

In recent studies, about 50% of patients have been noted to be asymptomatic at diagnosis.[3,8–12] An increasing number of children and adolescents are being diagnosed with AAOCA following routine preparticipation screening, presence of a murmur, or an abnormal electrocardiogram (ECG).[10,11] Typical presenting symptoms that have been reported are exertional chest pain, palpitations, syncope, as well as SCA.[11,12]

Transthoracic echocardiography (TTE) is the first-line imaging modality for the initial diagnosis.[13,14] Recent report by Lorber and colleagues, found variable agreement between TTE and surgical findings.[14] In another study, TTE reliably and prospectively diagnosed AAOCA in more than 95% of the cohort, and the echo findings were always consistent with the surgical descriptions of the anatomy.[10] Lorber and colleagues also suggested that, apart from the use of TTE in the diagnosis of the abnormal coronary origins, TTE can be helpful in identifying critical anatomic features such as intramural/interarterial course, which may influence surgical management. However, they demonstrated that the assessment of coronary ostium as well as intramyocardial course was not well delineated by TTE. Thus, advanced imaging modalities, including computed tomography angiography (CTA) or cardiac magnetic resonance imaging (CMR) are extremely helpful in comprehensively defining the anatomy of the AAOCA, including ostial morphology, interarterial, intramural, or intramyocardial course.[15–22]

Noninvasive Testing Under Provocative Stress

Exercise stress test. Exercise stress test (EST) is recommended in the evaluation of patients with coronary anomalies to assess for ischemic changes during exercise.[23,24] It has been used widely in children with coronary artery anomalies who can tolerate exercise, although it has a low sensitivity to detect inducible ischemia in this population.[5,10,23–29] Moreover, the interpretation of inducible ischemia may vary according to different studies when EST is reported "abnormal," which may reflect blunted blood pressure response, occurrence of premature ventricular contractions, or ST segment depression/elevation, the latter clearly with high specificity indicating inducible myocardial ischemia.[10,22,27,30] SCD during exertion has been reported in patients with coronary artery anomalies who had a normal EST before the event.[5] Brothers and colleagues reported a patient with AAOCA who initially had ischemic changes on EST but a repeat EST 1 week later was reassuring, which raised the question of intermittent nature of ischemia in the setting of AAOCA.[31] Current guidelines state that asymptomatic patients with AAORCA would be considered low-risk if EST is normal.[23,24] However,

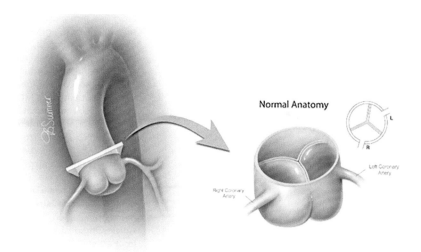

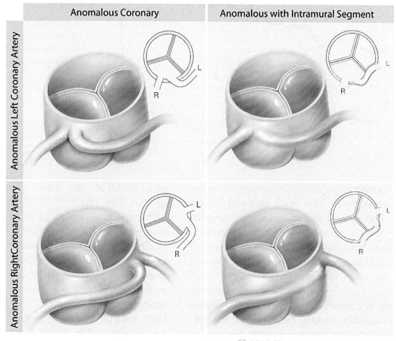

Fig. 1. Normal coronary anatomy and AAOCA subtypes. Used with permission of Texas Children's Hospital.

compelling data by Qasim and colleagues demonstrated the addition of cardiopulmonary exercise testing improved sensitivity of EST in patients with AAOCA, although EST is not well correlated with dobutamine stress CMR (DSCMR; Fig. 2).[26] Additionally, ischemic changes were recorded in only 1% of EST in a group of 164 patients with AAORCA.[25] Despite having a poor sensitivity, EST remains a valuable tool and seems to be specific in the presence of ST segment changes suggestive of myocardial ischemia. Continued data gathering and correlation with other provocative tests investigating inducible myocardial ischemia is needed to further define its role in this young population with AAOCA.

Stress echocardiography. Stress echocardiography has been established to identify new regional wall motion abnormalities or valvular dysfunction indicative of inducible myocardial ischemia following exercise (treadmill/cycloergometer) or during pharmacologic stress using dobutamine/atropine or adenosine/dipyridimole.[32–38] Heart rate decreases quickly, particularly in young children, a limitation that may prevent accurate acquisition and reading of

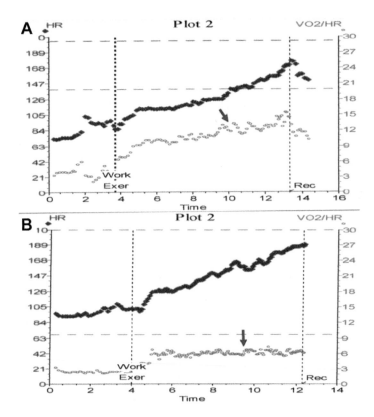

Fig. 2. Cardiopulmonary exercise testing (CPET) graphs showing normal upsloping O$_2$ pulse curve (*blue arrow*) (*A*) in a patient with AAORCA and abnormal flattening of O$_2$ pulse curve (*blue arrow*) (*B*) in a patient with AAORCA (patient also had subendocardial hypoperfusion in anterior and inferior septum on DSCMR). The horizontal dotted line on CPET graphs represents the maximal percentage predicted O$_2$ pulse for body mass. (*From* Qasim A, Doan TT, Pham TDN, Molossi S. Poster: Exercise stress testing in risk stratification of Anomalous Aortic Origin of a Coronary Artery. In: Pediatric Reseacrh Symposium at Texas Children's Hospital. ; 2021. https://www.texaschildrens.org/sites/default/files/uploads/documents/symposia/2021/posters/90.pdf. Printed with permission from Texas Children's Hospital.)

images. Pharmacologic stimuli, however, allow for sustained peak heart rate with optimal image acquisition during peak stress, including in smaller children or infants.[39] It is available in most centers, portable, and less expensive than other advanced imaging modalities. Notwithstanding, training and expertise is important in the assessment of regional wall motion abnormalities, which may limit its use in centers with low patient volume and/or with variable readers. Yet, stress echocardiography has been used in the pediatric population with a wide variety of indications where coronary lesions are suspected, such as acquired coronary disease and repaired/unrepaired congenital heart disease,[34,35,40,41] and as the preferred method to evaluate inducible myocardial ischemia in children/adolescents with AAOCA in some centers.[10,22,39,42–44] Currently, studies comparing different noninvasive testing modalities in the assessment of myocardial perfusion in AAOCA is lacking.

Advanced imaging on provocative stress

Nuclear perfusion imaging. Nuclear perfusion imaging (NPI) with provocative stress is well established in adults for the evaluation of coronary artery/ischemic heart disease. Its use in the evaluation of inducible ischemia in the young

with AAOCA has been reported by several groups (Fig. 3B).[22,27,30,44–47] However, concerns with patient exposure to ionizing radiation, high incidence of false-positive and false-negative findings, low spatial resolution, and attenuation artifacts are all factors that have resulted in decreasing interest for the use of NPI in this population. These are reasons that led our institution to transition to DSCMR as its safety, feasibility, and utility in a large cohort of children and adolescents with AAOCA have been recently published.[27,28,48–50]

Stress cardiac magnetic resonance imaging. Stress cardiac magnetic resonance imaging has been reported to improve patient outcome when used to guide revascularization decision in adults with ischemic heart disease.[51–60] Several studies have demonstrated its safety and feasibility in children with coronary artery involvement following a diagnosis of Kawasaki disease and repaired complex congenital heart disease that include coronary artery transfer (ie, following arterial switch operation).[61–65] In these studies, hyperemia was achieved using adenosine or its selective alpha-2A receptor agonist (Regadenoson) to potentially unmask fixed obstructive coronary

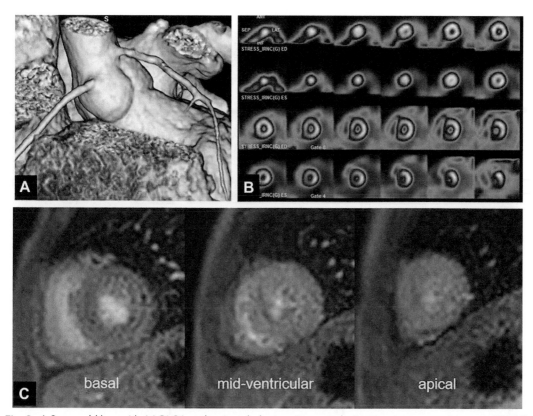

Fig. 3. A 9-year-old boy with AAOLCA at the sinotubular junction near the intercoronary commissure on CTA (A). Patient had a reassuring nuclear stress perfusion study (B), and no subendocardial hypoperfusion on DSCMR (C).

lesions. The proposed mechanism by which inducible ischemia may occur in patients with AAOCA has been postulated to relate to dynamic obstruction during exertion, although ostial abnormalities may be contributory as a fixed mechanism. Dobutamine has been viewed to closely mimic exercise because it increases contractility and decreases systemic vascular resistance,[56,57,65,66] thus inducing wall motion abnormalities at a time of maximal myocardial oxygen demand. DSCMR has demonstrated excellent performance with good prediction of ischemic events in adults.[54,66,67] First-pass perfusion, in addition to assessment of wall motion abnormalities, has increased the sensitivity of DSCMR, in keeping with the mechanism in demand ischemia cascade (where impaired perfusion precedes wall motion abnormalities).[56–58,60] Stress CMR additionally provides high-quality cardiac imaging with excellent spatial resolution and avoids ionizing radiation, an important factor especially in children/adolescents.[68–71] Doan and colleagues reported the largest cohort of children with AAOCA undergoing DSCMR,[48] including 224 studies in 182 patients younger than 20 years and median age of 14 years. Most studies were successfully completed with no sedation and 99% were free of major events, with only 12.5% reported minor events (Fig. 3; Fig. 4). Inducible perfusion defects were seen in 14%, and 42% among these had associated wall motion abnormalities. This study demonstrated safety and feasibility of DSCMR in the young patient with AAOCA and greatly contributed to management decisions.[48] Moreover, agreement between DSCMR and invasive fractional flow reserve (FFR) during dobutamine challenge was demonstrated in 13 young patients with AAOCA.[72] Comparable data was demonstrated in isolated case reports and intraseptal AAOLCA in a cohort of 19 patients reported by Doan and colleagues.[73–75] These authors reported stress perfusion imaging studies in 14 patients and 50% had inducible perfusion defects.[75] Given these more recent data, DSCMR clearly seems to have a defining role for the detection of perfusion abnormalities in AAOCA, allowing for comparison of results after surgical repair (in those patients for whom this intervention is indicated) with resolution of the inducible ischemia determined postoperatively (see Fig. 4).[27,28,48,49] However, image quality and expertise are paramount for the

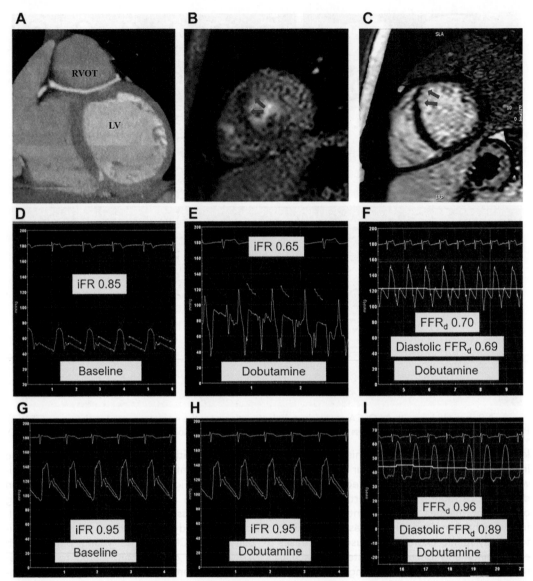

Fig. 4. A 16-year-old male patient with recurrent chest pain during wrestling practice. CTA showed AAOLCA with intraseptal course of the LCA (A). DSCMR showed subendocardial hypoperfusion in the anteroseptal wall (*red arrows*) (B), and late-gadolinium enhancement (*red arrows*) (C) indicates inducible ischemia and likely history of subendocardial infarction. Baseline iFR <0.89 (D), which further decreased to 0.65 (E), and diastolic FFR 0.69 <0.80 (F) consistent with impaired coronary flow. Following supraarterial myotomy of the intraseptal segment through a right ventriculotomy and direct reimplantation of the LCA, there were normalization of baseline iFR to 0.95 (G); at peak dobutamine stress, normal values of iFR at 0.95 (H), FFR at 0.96, and diastolic FFR at 0.89 (I). (*From* Doan TT, Molossi S, Qureshi AM, McKenzie ED. Intraseptal Anomalous Coronary Artery With Myocardial Infarction: Novel Surgical Approach. Ann Thorac Surg. 2020 Oct;110(4):e271-e274.)

visual assessment of first-pass perfusion of gadolinium, specifically to differentiate dark rim artifacts from a true inducible perfusion defect. Risk stratification in AAOCA continues to be a challenge to determine those patients at risk for myocardial ischemia and DSCMR is clearly contributing to decision-making in this population.

Invasive Testing Under Provocative Stress Angiography. Angiography is generally not the first choice of imaging to diagnose anomalous coronary arteries in children. However, it is part of invasive assessment of coronary artery flow and has been performed in recent years when there is conflict between clinical data and results from noninvasive studies.[76,77] Using pharmacologic stressors to mimic physiologic changes that occur during exercise may disclose hemodynamically significant lesions that would benefit from intervention, including measurement of coronary flow and angiographic assessment of the vessel diameter (Fig. 5B, C).

Fractional flow reserve. FFR is a pressure-derived index of severity in the setting of coronary artery stenosis, calculated as a ratio between mean intracoronary pressure distal to the lesion (Pd) and mean aortic pressure (Pa) obtained during the entire cardiac cycle (see Fig. 4; Fig. 5). It requires the use of a coronary vasodilator to unmask a fixed obstructive coronary lesion. In adults with ischemic heart disease, coronary revascularization is typically indicated with FFR less than 0.8. In the setting of dynamic mechanisms leading to coronary compression, such as in AAOCA with intramural course or intraseptal course, dobutamine is considered the preferred pharmacologic agent to induce provocative stress mimicking some physiologic changes that occur with exercise.[48,65,78] Dobutamine induces positive inotropy and increased cardiac output, as it also induces decrease in systemic and coronary vascular resistance.[79–81] Diastolic FFR (dFFR), however, might constitute a better indicator of intracoronary hemodynamic assessment during dobutamine infusion given a potential overshooting of distal systolic pressure, which in turn may nullify a significant diastolic pressure gradient.[82] The initial data on the use of FFR in children with AAOCA was presented by Agrawal and colleagues in 2017, although in a small cohort that included 4 patients with AAOCA, stating its contribution in risk stratification in select patients.[76] As dFFR is calculated manually (average of 3 Pd/Pa ratio using digital calipers at end systole), it comprises a major limitation. In addition, the use of dobutamine is contraindicated in patients presenting with SCA, further limiting the assessment of FFR in AAOCA.

Instantaneous wave-free ratio. Instantaneous wave-free ratio (iFR) is a drug-free pressure-derived index of coronary artery flow during a period of naturally constant and low resistance due to minimal competing pressure waves in diastole (see Figs. 4 and 5).[83] In theory, advantages of this index include no need of a vasodilator to reduce coronary vascular resistance and better procedure tolerance due to shorter procedure time.[84] iFR showed better agreement with coronary flow velocity reserve when compared with (JUSTIFY-CFR study)[85] and noninferior to FFR because it relates to health outcomes in guiding coronary revascularization in adults with ischemic heart disease.[84,86] Doan and colleagues very recently first reported the use of iFR in children with AAOCA.[78] Data showed that iFR correlated with adenosine FFR and dobutamine dFFR, thus being an alternative to those patients in which pharmacologic stressors (eg, dobutamine) are contraindicated. Moreover, the authors stated the data contributed to decision-making regarding coronary

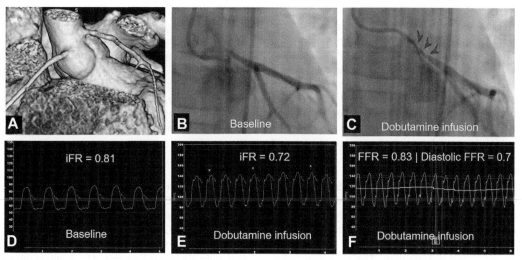

Fig. 5. Angiogram and intracoronary hemodynamic assessment in a 9-year-old boy with AAOLCA at the sinotubular junction near the intercoronary commissure on CTA (A). Despite reassuring DSCMR and nuclear stress perfusion study (see Fig. 3), the proximal LCA caliber changed from subtle narrowing (B) to severely compressed (*red arrowheads*) during dobutamine infusion (C). Baseline iFR <0.89 indicates significant coronary artery compression (D) and iFR further reduced during dobutamine infusion (E). Diastolic FFR <0.8 consistent with significant coronary flow impairment during provocative testing with dobutamine (F).

intervention. Additional recent data from the same authors published resting iFR and dFFR with dobutamine challenge guiding decision-making in a subset of patients with concerning clinical symptoms but negative noninvasive perfusion studies under provocative stress.[87] These abnormal values of intracoronary flow were shown to completely resolve on repeat invasive studies following surgical intervention (see Fig. 4G–I).

Of interest, the principles of iFR during dobutamine challenge neutralizes the systolic overshooting phenomenon in the assessment of potential dynamic compression in AAOCA, indicating that dynamic compression during provocative stress could be of value in unfolding hemodynamic significant coronary obstruction in the setting of AAOCA. Specifically, Ghobrial and colleagues published their center experience in symptomatic adult AAOCA patients using iFR and dobutamine challenge.[88] Similarly, these authors reported improvement in dobutamine iFR in 18 patients following surgical repair of the anomalous vessel. We have observed similar pattern of provocative pharmacologic stress with dobutamine affect iFR values in children with AAOCA compared with those seen at rest in our center (unpublished data). As promising as these data on significant improvement in iFR and FFR following surgical repair of AAOCA are,[89] it is important to keep in perspective that such cutoff values derive from ischemic coronary artery disease in adults and may not be the optimal values in the setting of AAOCA, which likely includes mostly a dynamic component leading to myocardial ischemia and sudden events, especially in the young population.

Intravascular ultrasound. Intravascular ultrasound (IVUS) in AAOCA has been widely used in adults and considered the gold standard for the assessment of the intramural segment given its excellent spatial determination and evaluation of dynamic lateral compression at rest and compared with pharmacologic stress.[4,90–92] Angelini and colleagues published data in adult patients with AAORCA where IVUS showed the worst area of stenosis in the intramural segment of the RCA proximally, immediately distal to its ostium.[90] IVUS performed under pharmacologic stress includes administration of saline bolus, atropine, and dobutamine. The diameter (minimal and maximal) of the anomalous coronary in the compromised area is measured in both systole and diastole. Significant coronary compression includes an area ratio greater than 50% at baseline and/or greater than 60% during

provocative stress.[90] Its use has also guided stent placement in the proximal intramural segment in select adults patients with AAORCA.[90] Although IVUS is used in pediatric patients for the evaluation of certain congenital heart lesions,[93] its use in the setting of AAOCA is hardly existent. Agrawal and colleagues reported a small cohort of pediatric patients with AAOCA and myocardial bridges describing the feasibility and safety of IVUS, and its significant contribution in management decision-making.[76] This seems promising in a very selected group of patients with AAOCA but substantial data are needed to determine its role in risk stratification in young patients. More importantly, perhaps, this should not be considered a common technique in the evaluation of young patients with AAOCA because expertise is essential to mitigate potential serious coronary complications with the procedure.

Management decision-making
Medical Management
At our institution, we use a previously published standardized approach in the assessment and management of AAOCA (Fig. 6).[27] Clinical follow-up without medication or intervention is indicated when the provocative testing is negative for ischemic changes in the asymptomatic patient with AAORCA.[94] Exercise restriction with or without beta-blocker therapy (in the setting of intraseptal AAOLCA) is indicated when surgery is recommended in a patient with AAOCA but surgery is either denied or not feasible given the anatomy.[73] In our experience, medical management in a young athlete with beta-blocker therapy is challenging given its effect in athletic performance. Therefore, surgical intervention is favored when it outweighs the risks. Following surgical repair of the anomalous coronary artery, we empirically recommend antiplatelet therapy with aspirin for 3 months, with discontinuation following reassuring postoperative studies at this time.

Surgical Approach
To date, the exact mechanisms of ischemia leading to SCA in AAOCA remain undefined, as do clinical and morphologic features that increase the risk of ischemia and SCA.[95–98] Surgical repair of AAOCA has been performed to potentially address this risk and mitigate the occurrence of SCA, although surgical indications and benefits remain unclear with significant variation in practice.[10,12,28,49,99,100] Current consensus guidelines provide a standardized approach that surgical intervention is recommended for those with signs and/or symptoms of

Clinical algorithm for patients with anomalous aortic origin or course of a coronary artery

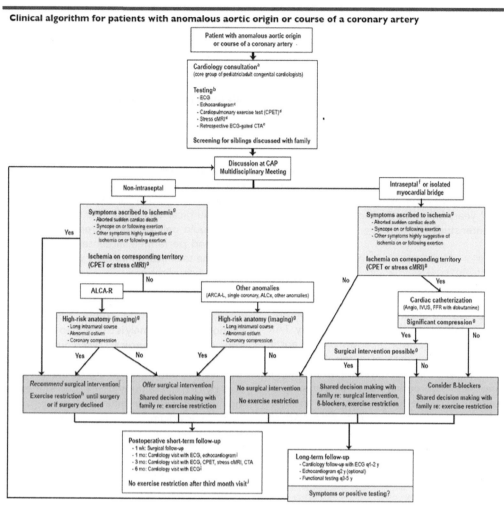

Fig. 6. Clinical algorithm for patients with anomalous aortic origin of a coronary artery.ALCA-R, anomalous left coronary from the right sinus; ALCx, anomalous left circumflex artery; ARCA-L, anomalous right coronary from the left sinus; CAP, coronary anomalies program. [a]Consent abtained for participation in prospective CHSS aand TCH databases. [b]Additional studies (Holter,cardiac catheterization, etc) may be performed depending on the clinical assessment.[c]External echocardiograms do not need to be repeated if the study is deemed appropriate. [d]CPET or stress cMRI not necessary on patients that present with aborted sudden cardiac death. These studies may be deferred in young patients. [e]An external CTA may be used if able to upload the images and the study provides all necessary information to make a decision. CTA should ne deferred in patients <8 years unless clinical concerns. [f]An intraseptal coronaru is as an abnormal vessel(usually a left coronary arising from the right sinus)that travels posteriorly into the septum below the level of the pulmonary valve. [g]Unrollfing if significant intramural segment, neo-ostium creation or voronary translocation if intramural segment behind a commissure,coronary translocation if short or no intramural segment. Surgical intervention will be offered for patients between 10 and 35 years of age. Other patients will be considered on a case-by-case basis. Aspirin will be administered for 3 months after surgery. [h]Restriction form participation in all competitive sports and in exercise with moderate or high dynamic component(> 40% maximal oxygen uptake-e.g.,soccer, tennis, swimming, basketball, American football). (Mitchell et al, JACC 2005:1364-1367). [i]Patient may be seen by outside primary cardiologist. [j]Postoperative patients will be cleared for exercise and competitive sports based on findings at the third month postoperative visit including results of CPET, stress cMRI and CTA. Used with permission of Texas Children's Hospital.

ischemia (class I).[23,24,94] In asymptomatic patients with reassuring diagnostic testing, surgery is recommended (class IIa) for patients with AAORCA who had ventricular arrhythmia and in AAOLCA.[94] Patients who are diagnosed with AAORCA can be considered for surgery despite reassuring testing and no other clinical concern (class IIb).[94] The goals of AAOCA repair are to yield an unobstructed coronary artery from the appropriate aortic sinus while minimizing the risk of procedural complications.[28,101] Surgical repair of AAOCA should aim at eliminating the intramural course and its associated ostial narrowing by unroofing, ostioplasty, or transection and reimplantation (TAR).[24] Unroofing of an intramural course is most commonly reported, although other techniques including TAR or neo-ostium creation have also been performed.[10,28,49,99,102,103] Repositioning of the pulmonary artery confluence away from the anomalous artery may be considered as an adjunctive procedure but less widely used.[24] Surgical intervention is generally successful, although complication and reoperation due to coronary artery stenosis have been reported up to 5% in the 7 years following the index operation in a multicenter study.[99]

Anomalous aortic origin of a coronary artery with interarterial course or anomalous aortic origin of the left coronary artery from the noncoronary sinus. The primary surgical strategies described at our center included unroofing of an intramural course and coronary TAR (Fig. 7). We do not favor takedown of the aortic commissure at the time of surgical unroofing due to the potential risk of postoperative aortic insufficiency.[28] Unroofing has been our surgical procedure of choice for patients with an intramural segment above the aortic valve in which the technique is believed to move the ostium to the correct sinus. TAR has been used for patients with short intramural length and the intramural segment traveling below the level of the

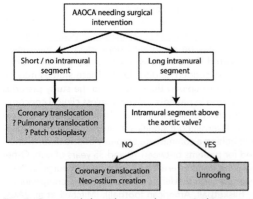

Fig. 7. Proposed algorithm to select surgical intervention techniques for patients with AAOCA based on coronary artery anatomy using computerized tomography angiography and surgical inspection. (*From* Mery CM, De León LE, Molossi S, Sexson-Tejtel SK, Agrawal H, Krishnamurthy R, Masand P, Qureshi AM, McKenzie ED, Fraser CD Jr. Outcomes of surgical intervention for anomalous aortic origin of a coronary artery: A large contemporary prospective cohort study. J Thorac Cardiovasc Surg. 2018 Jan;155(1):305-319.e4.)

aortic valve commissure, in whom surgical unroofing would not result in placing the ostium in its correct aortic sinus (Fig. 8).[28,49,101]

Coronary unroofing is a widely used technique and is considered relatively safe in the surgical repair of AAOCA.[10,103–106] Coronary TAR has been performed in both adults and children when the unroofing technique is deemed to have potential disruption of the aortic valve integrity.[49,100,107,108] TAR requires extensive coronary manipulation involving transection followed by reimplantation of the anomalous coronary artery without an aortic button. It is important to emphasize that it is still unknown which surgical technique is superior, and that TAR should only be considered in select candidates and performed in centers with expertise given the technical complexity with potential iatrogenic complications.[109]

Anomalous aortic origin of the left coronary artery with intraseptal course. Surgical intervention for this anomaly is challenged by the limitation of current surgical techniques and the uncertainty of long-term outcomes. Najm and colleagues performed unroofing of the intraseptal LCA by circumferentially transecting and extending the right ventricular infundibulum using autologous pericardium.[110,111] The authors reported excellent surgical outcome in 14 patients who have been followed between 1.5 and 45 months.[111] Others have reported anterior translocation of the right pulmonary artery and division of the muscle overlying the LCA externally between the aortic root and pulmonary artery.[12] We have reported a successful supraarterial myotomy of the intraseptal segment through a right ventriculotomy and direct reimplantation of the left coronary artery. This patient recovered well with improved physiologic provocative testing following surgery and has returned to competitive wrestling without issues.[74]

Recommendations to physical activities
Consensus guidelines state that individuals with AAOCA and symptoms of ischemic chest pain or syncope suspected to be due to ventricular arrhythmias, or a history of aborted SCD, should be activity restricted and offered surgery.[24] The asymptomatic patient with AAORCA and no evidence of ischemia clinically and with provocative testing can participate in competitive athletics. However, patients and family should be appropriately informed and counseled of the known risk of SCD, although rare, and the uncertain accuracy of a negative stress test.[23] It is important to recommend preparedness for cardiac events such as

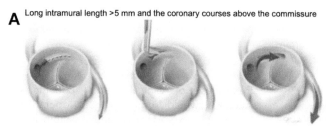

A Long intramural length >5 mm and the coronary courses above the commissure

Surgical unroofing of the intramural segment

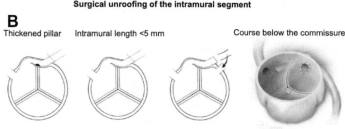

B

Thickened pillar   Intramural length <5 mm   Course below the commissure

Transection and Reimplantation

Fig. 8. Diagrams of surgical unroofing of an intramural course (*A*) versus transection and reimplantation (*B*) based on anatomic features on CTA and surgical inspection. Used with permission of Texas Children's Hospital.

having an automated external defibrillator (AED) available with individuals who know how to use it, as part of an emergency action plan. However, individuals with untreated AAOLCA from the opposite (right) anterior sinus of Valsalva, regardless of symptomatology, are restricted from all competitive sports.[23,24,94]

Following successful surgical repair of AAOCA, athletes may consider participation in all sports 3 months after surgery if the patient remains free of symptoms, an EST shows no evidence of ischemia or cardiac arrhythmias, and a stress perfusion imaging study shows no inducible perfusion defect or regional wall motion abnormalities.[24,27,28] In patients who presented with aborted SCD, a longer postoperative period (12 months) may be necessary to ensure patients are free of symptoms suggesting ischemia or arrhythmia and have no evidence of myocardial ischemia on provocative testing or concerning arrhythmia.[24] An AED should be available for all of these patients with available personnel who are trained in cardiopulmonary resuscitation and how to use an AED.[24]

ANOMALOUS CORONARY ARTERY ORIGIN FROM THE PULMONARY ARTERY
Prevalence, Anatomy, Physiology, and Diagnosis
Prevalence
Anomalous origin of the left coronary artery from pulmonary artery (ALCAPA) is a rare disease, occurring in 1 in 3,00,000 live births or 0.4% of patients with congenital cardiac abnormalities,[112] that if untreated causes heart failure, myocardial ischemia, and death. The incidence

of ALCAPA is thought to be higher than that of anomalous origin of the right coronary artery from pulmonary artery (ARCAPA) due to the proximity of the left coronary bud to the pulmonary artery sinus (although ARCAPA may have been underdiagnosed due to its initially relatively innocuous nature compared with ALCAPA).[113,114] ARCAPA is known to occur in 0.002% of patients with congenital cardiac abnormalities.[114–116]

Anatomy
The most common defect of this type is ALCAPA, sometimes known as Bland-White-Garland syndrome.[117,118] In some cases, the left anterior descending and left circumflex coronary arteries have individual origins from the pulmonary artery, with similar pathophysiologic and clinical sequelae.[119,120] The origin of the right coronary artery from the pulmonary artery has been thought to be benign; however, clinical sequelae have been described although later in life.[121]

Physiology
Fetuses with ALCAPA remain asymptomatic because the diastolic pressure in the pulmonary artery and aorta are similar during prenatal circulation. When the pulmonary vascular resistance starts to drop after birth, symptoms start to appear in most infants due to a reversal flow through left coronary artery. This leads to coronary artery steal and further progression of myocardial ischemia. This may be exacerbated during periods of stress, which in infants can occur during feedings. The surrounding arteries start to create collateral blood flow to the

affected ventricle. Mitral valve regurgitation occurs in the disease process secondary to ventricular dilatation and papillary muscle ischemia. Patients may initially present with subtle symptoms of extreme fussiness with feeds, due to the ischemia, and ultimately progress toward respiratory distress as heart failure ensues.[122–124] Nevertheless, many patients may do well and be completely asymptomatic, engaging in sports activities until late childhood and adolescence when the diagnosis is established following evaluation for a murmur (commonly mitral regurgitation from chronic ischemia to the mitral valve apparatus).

Due to the reduced ventricular workload and oxygen demands of the right ventricle compared with that of the left ventricle, ventricular ischemia is less prominent in ARCAPA than in ALCAPA and may present in adult life. However, ARCAPA patients with a right dominant coronary circulation do exhibit chronic ischemia and have increased adverse outcomes than patients with a left dominant circulation.[125,126]

Diagnosis

This condition is usually suspected on echocardiography either by direct visualization of the coronary artery from the pulmonary artery or by secondary signs of ventricular dysfunction, mitral regurgitation, echogenic papillary muscles, dilation of right coronary artery (due to collateral formation in ALCAPA) as well as the presence of flow signals within the myocardium suggesting collateral flow (Figs. 9 and 10).[127,128] Noninvasive cross-sectional imaging with either CTA or CMR may assist in more definitive diagnosis and provide additional information.

The electrocardiogram of a patient with ALCAPA may show evidence for anterolateral ischemia or infarction, including transient or chronic ST-segment changes in the anterolateral leads or Q waves in leads I aVL, V5, and V6.[129]

Although patients with ARCAPA may mirror the symptoms of ALCAPA, it is usually diagnosed at autopsy or in asymptomatic children or adults. Electrocardiographic findings are often nonspecific. The diagnosis can be made with careful TTE that includes meticulous attention to the origins of the coronary arteries. CTA of the coronary arteries is also diagnostic. Alternatively, cardiac catheterization provides hemodynamic assessment in addition to coronary angiography to confirm the diagnosis.[114,116,130]

Surgical Approach

All anomalously originating coronary arteries from the pulmonary artery require surgical correction. At this time, there are no percutaneous treatment options to repair this anomaly.

Anomalous origin of the left coronary artery from the pulmonary artery

Regardless of clinical status, patients with ALCAPA would require urgent operation.[130] Creating a two-artery coronary system is indicated in all situations, including critically ill infants. Available pathologic information indicates that either a tunnel (Takeuchi) repair or translocation of the connection to the aortic root, if feasible.[130] Takeuchi described the procedure involving creation of a coronary tunnel inside the pulmonary artery to establish continuity between the aorta and the LCA ostium, in 1979.[131–133] This procedure was useful in cases in which direct implantation was thought to be difficult because of unfavorable coronary anatomy. Use of this method is declining given the high rate of complications including supravalvular pulmonary stenosis, intrapulmonary baffle leaks, and aortic valve insufficiency as well as a 30% chance of reoperation or catheter intervention over time. Thus, direct reimplantation has increasingly become the procedure of choice. Urgent corrective surgery to establish a two-coronary circulation is shown to lead to quick recovery of ventricular function in majority with excellent long-term survival.[131,134–137] A recent cohort study by Patel and colleagues described early surgical outcomes in 37 subjects with ALCAPA with short length of postoperative stay, low morbidity, and no surgical mortality. As in prior studies, they found more late complications with the Takeuchi procedure compared with direct reimplantation.[128] These patients had excellent status at their long-term follow-up, with a significant improvement in the left ventricular ejection fraction and mitral valve regurgitation.[128,138,139] Despite normal ejection fraction, most patients had abnormal measurement of myocardial mechanics.[138]

Anomalous origin of the right coronary artery from the pulmonary artery

According to the latest American Heart Association/American College of Cardiology guidelines, repair is a Class I recommendation for symptomatic patients with ARCAPA and a Class IIa recommendation in asymptomatic patients with ventricular dysfunction or myocardial ischemia attributed to ARCAPA.[94] Surgical intervention consists of reimplantation of the RCA, including excising the anomalous origin of the RCA along with a button of the pulmonary arterial wall and

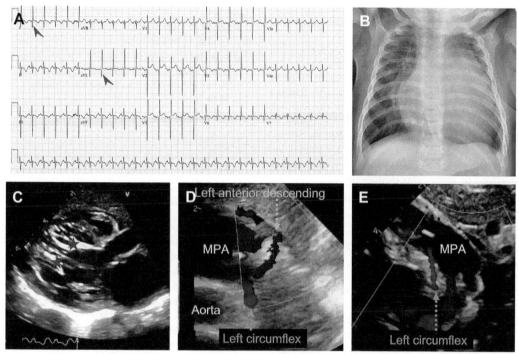

Fig. 9. ALCAPA in a 2-month-old infant who presented with failure to thrive and heart failure. ECG showed normal sinus rhythm, left axis deviation, Q wave in lead I and aVL (*arrowheads*), and T-wave inversion in the inferolateral leads (*A*), severe cardiomegaly and pulmonary edema (*B*), echogenic papillary muscles (*red stars, C*), retrograde flow in the left anterior descending coronary artery (*D*), and circumflex artery (*E*). MPA, main pulmonary artery.

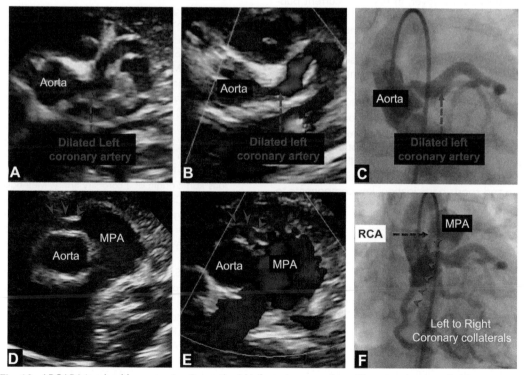

Fig. 10. ARCAPA in a healthy appearing 9-month-old infant who was referred for an evaluation of a heart murmur. Echocardiographic images demonstrated dilated left coronary artery with normal aortic origin and prograde flow (*A–C*), which then provides flow to the right coronary artery (RCA, *arrowheads*), which connects to the main pulmonary artery (MPA) with flow from RCA to MPA (*D–F*).

translocating it into the anterior aspect of the ascending aorta.[114,130]

Recommendations to physical activities
Athletes with ALCAPA or ARCAPA can participate only in low-intensity class IA sports, whether or not they have had a prior myocardial infarction, and pending repair of the anomaly.[23] After repair of ALCAPA and ARCAPA, decisions regarding exercise restriction may be based on the presence of sequelae such as myocardial infarction or ventricular dysfunction.[23]

SUMMARY

Congenital coronary anomalies are not an infrequent occurrence, and their clinical presentation typically occurs during early years, although may be manifested only in adulthood. In the setting of AAOCA, this is particularly concerning because it inflicts sudden loss of healthy young lives. This event, although rare, leads to incalculable grief in families, organizations, and communities. An anomalous origin of one or more coronary arteries from the pulmonary artery is hemodynamically significant and produces myocardial ischemia leading to ischemic cardiomyopathy or SCD, thus surgical intervention in this setting is well defined. However, in AAOCA, current published consensus guidelines for the diagnosis and management of these abnormalities are limited by insufficient evidence due to lack of hard endpoints. There remains significant variability in risk stratification and management decisions, particularly in the asymptomatic patient. Standardized approach to the evaluation of these patients, with careful data collection and collaboration among centers, is likely the way to improve risk stratification and lead to optimal management decision. Such strategies will foster a safer environment for these patients to engage in exercise and sports participation, key components to successful and healthier lives.

CLINICS CARE POINTS

- Coronary artery anomalies may occur in up to 1% of the population and comprise the second most frequent cause of sudden death in the young.
- Echocardiography can diagnose up to 95% of patients, though advanced imaging is essential to define morphologic features.
- Myocardial functional studies under provocative stress are important in risk stratification.

- Surgical intervention may be indicated in a subset of patients.
- Exercise activities should be carefully considered as sedentarism is a great risk factor for lifetime cardiovascular disease.

DISCLOSURE

The authors have nothing to disclose.

REFERENCES

1. Angelini P, Velasco JA, Flamm S. Coronary anomalies: incidence, pathophysiology, and clinical relevance. Circulation 2002;105(20):2449–54.
2. Kayalar N, Burkhart HM, Dearani JA, et al. Congenital coronary anomalies and surgical treatment. Congenit Heart Dis 2009;4(4):239–51.
3. Maron BJ, Doerer JJ, Haas TS, et al. Sudden deaths in young competitive athletes analysis of 1866 deaths in the United States, 1980-2006. Circulation 2009;119(8):1085–92.
4. Angelini P. Coronary artery anomalies: an entity in search of an identity. Circulation 2007;115(10):1296–305.
5. Basso C, Maron BJ, Corrado D, et al. Clinical profile of congenital coronary artery anomalies with origin from the wrong aortic sinus leading to sudden death in young competitive athletes. J Am Coll Cardiol 2000;35(6):1493–501.
6. Cheezum M, O'Gara P, Blankstein R, et al. Anomalous aortic origin of a coronary artery from the inappropriate sinus of Valsalva. J Am Coll Cardiol 2017;69(12). https://doi.org/10.1016/j.jacc.2017.01.031.
7. Molossi S, Sachdeva S. Anomalous coronary arteries. Curr Opin Cardiol 2020;35(1):42–51.
8. Molossi S, Martínez-Bravo LE, Mery CM. Anomalous aortic origin of a coronary artery. Methodist Debakey Cardiovasc J 2017;15(2):111–21.
9. Mainwaring RD, Reddy VM, Reinhartz O, et al. Surgical repair of anomalous aortic origin of a coronary artery. Eur J Cardio-thoracic Surg 2014;46(1):20–6.
10. Sachdeva S, Frommelt MA, Mitchell ME, et al. Surgical unroofing of intramural anomalous aortic origin of a coronary artery in pediatric patients: single-center perspective. J Thorac Cardiovasc Surg 2018;155(4):1760–8.
11. Molossi S, Agrawal H. Clinical evaluation of anomalous aortic origin of a coronary artery (AAOCA). Congenit Heart Dis 2017;12(5):607–9.
12. Mainwaring RD, Murphy DJ, Rogers IS, et al. Surgical repair of 115 patients with anomalous aortic origin of a coronary artery from a single

institution. World J Pediatr Congenit Hear Surg 2016;7(3):353–9.

13. Frommelt PC, Berger S, Pelech AN, et al. Prospective identification of anomalous origin of left coronary artery from the right sinus of Valsalva using transthoracic echocardiography: importance of color Doppler flow mapping. Pediatr Cardiol 2001;22(4):327–32.

14. Lorber R, Srivastava S, Wilder TJ, et al. Anomalous aortic origin of coronary arteries in the young echocardiographic evaluation with surgical correlation. JACC Cardiovasc Imaging 2015;8(11): 1239–49.

15. de Jonge GJ, van Ooijen PMA, Piers LH, et al. Visualization of anomalous coronary arteries on dual-source computed tomography. Eur Radiol 2008;18(11):2425–32.

16. Kacmaz F, Ozbulbul NI, Alyan O, et al. Imaging of coronary artery anomalies: the role of multidetector computed tomography. Coron Artery Dis 2008;19(3):203–9.

17. Komatsu S, Sato Y, Ichikawa M, et al. Anomalous coronary arteries in adults detected by multislice computed tomography: presentation of cases from multicenter registry and review of the literature. Heart Vessels 2008;23(1):26–34.

18. Lee S, Uppu SC, Lytrivi ID, et al. Utility of multimodality imaging in the morphologic characterization of anomalous aortic origin of a coronary artery. World J Pediatr Congenit Heart Surg 2016;7(3):308–17.

19. Su JT, Chung T, Muthupillai R, et al. Usefulness of real-time navigator magnetic resonance imaging for evaluating coronary artery origins in pediatric patients. Am J Cardiol 2005;95(5):679–82.

20. Aljaroudi WA, Flamm SD, Saliba W, et al. Role of CMR imaging in risk stratification for sudden cardiac death. JACC Cardiovasc Imaging 2013;6(3): 392–406.

21. Brothers JA, Whitehead KK, Keller MS, et al. Cardiac MRI and CT: differentiation of normal ostium and intraseptal course from slitlike ostium and interarterial course in anomalous left coronary artery in children. AJR Am J Roentgenol 2015;204(1): W104–9.

22. Brothers JA, McBride MG, Seliem MA, et al. Evaluation of myocardial ischemia after surgical repair of anomalous aortic origin of a coronary artery in a series of pediatric patients. J Am Coll Cardiol 2007;50(21):2078–82.

23. Van Hare GF, Ackerman MJ, Evangelista J-AK, et al. Eligibility and disqualification recommendations for competitive athletes with cardiovascular abnormalities: task force 4: congenital heart disease: a scientific statement from the American heart association and American College of Cardiology. Circulation 2015;132(22):e281–91.

24. Brothers JA, Frommelt MA, Jaquiss RDB, et al. Expert consensus guidelines: anomalous aortic origin of a coronary artery. J Thorac Cardiovasc Surg 2017;153(6):1440–57.

25. Doan TT, Bonilla-ramirez C, Sachdeva S, et al. Abstract 13007 : myocardial ischemia in anomalous aortic origin of a right coronary artery : medium-term follow-up in a large prospective cohort. Circulation 2020;142(suppl_3):A13007.

26. Qasim A, Doan TT, Pham TD, et al. Is exercise stress testing useful for risk stratification in anomalous aortic origin of a coronary artery? Semin Thorac Cardiovasc Surg 2022. In press.

27. Molossi S, Agrawal H, Mery CM, et al. Outcomes in anomalous aortic origin of a coronary artery following a prospective standardized approach. Circ Cardiovasc Interv 2020;13(2):e008445.

28. Mery CM, De León LE, Molossi S, et al. Outcomes of surgical intervention for anomalous aortic origin of a coronary artery: a large contemporary prospective cohort study. J Thorac Cardiovasc Surg 2018;155(1):305–19.e4.

29. Maeda K, Schnittger I, Murphy DJ, et al. Surgical unroofing of hemodynamically significant myocardial bridges in a pediatric population. J Thorac Cardiovasc Surg 2018;156(4):1618–26.

30. Cho S-H, Joo H-C, Yoo K-J, et al. Anomalous origin of right coronary artery from left coronary sinus: surgical management and clinical result. Thorac Cardiovasc Surg 2015;63(5):360–6.

31. Brothers J, Carter C, McBride M, et al. Anomalous left coronary artery origin from the opposite sinus of Valsalva: evidence of intermittent ischemia. J Thorac Cardiovasc Surg 2010;140(2):e27–9.

32. Paridon SM, Alpert BS, Boas SR, et al. Clinical stress testing in the pediatric age group: a statement from the American Heart Association council on cardiovascular disease in the young, committee on atherosclerosis, hypertension, and obesity in youth. Circulation 2006;113(15):1905–20.

33. Pellikka PA, Arruda-Olson A, Chaudhry FA, et al. Guidelines for performance, interpretation, and application of stress echocardiography in ischemic heart disease: from the American society of echocardiography. J Am Soc Echocardiogr 2020;33(1):1–41. e8.

34. Chen MH, Abernathey E, Lunze F, et al. Utility of exercise stress echocardiography in pediatric cardiac transplant recipients: a single-center experience. J Hear Lung Transpl 2012;31(5):517–23.

35. El Assaad I, Gauvreau K, Rizwan R, et al. Value of exercise stress echocardiography in children with hypertrophic cardiomyopathy. J Am Soc Echocardiogr 2020;33(7):888–94.e2.

36. Badruddin SM, Ahmad A, Mickelson J, et al. Supine bicycle versus post-treadmill exercise echocardiography in the detection of myocardial

ischemia: a randomized single-blind crossover trial. J Am Coll Cardiol 1999;33(6):1485–90.

37. Kimball TR. Pediatric stress echocardiography. Pediatr Cardiol 2002;23(3):347–57.

38. Armstrong WF, Zoghbi WA. Stress echocardiography: current methodology and clinical applications. J Am Coll Cardiol 2005;45(11):1739–47.

39. Thompson WR. Stress echocardiography in paediatrics: implications for the evaluation of anomalous aortic origin of the coronary arteries. Cardiol Young 2015;25(8):1524–30.

40. Pahl E, Duffy CE, Chaudhry FA. The role of stress echocardiography in children. Echocardiography 2000;17(5):507–12.

41. Ou P, Kutty S, Khraiche D, et al. Acquired coronary disease in children: the role of multimodality imaging. Pediatr Radiol 2013;43(4):444–53.

42. Deng ES, O'Brien SE, Fynn-Thompson F, et al. Recurrent sudden cardiac arrests in a child with an anomalous left coronary artery. JACC Case Rep 2021;3(13):1527–30.

43. Lameijer H, Kampman MAM, Oudijk MA, et al. Ischaemic heart disease during pregnancy or post-partum: systematic review and case series. Neth Hear J 2015;23(5):249–57.

44. Fabozzo A, DiOrio M, Newburger JW, et al. Anomalous aortic origin of coronary arteries: a single-center experience. Semin Thorac Cardiovasc Surg 2016;28(4):791–800.

45. Mumtaz MA, Lorber RE, Arruda J, et al. Surgery for anomalous aortic origin of the coronary artery. Ann Thorac Surg 2011;91(3):811–5.

46. Agati S, Secinaro A, Caldaroni F, et al. Perfusion study helps in the management of the intraseptal course of an anomalous coronary artery. World J Pediatr Congenit Hear Surg 2019;10(3):360–3.

47. Blomjous MSH, Budde RPJ, Bekker MWA, et al. Clinical outcome of anomalous coronary artery with interarterial course in adults: single-center experience combined with a systematic review. Int J Cardiol 2021;335:32–9.

48. Doan TT, Molossi S, Sachdeva S, et al. Dobutamine stress cardiac MRI is safe and feasible in pediatric patients with anomalous aortic origin of a coronary artery (AAOCA). Int J Cardiol 2021; 334:42–8.

49. Bonilla-Ramirez C, Molossi S, Sachdeva S, et al. Outcomes in anomalous aortic origin of a coronary artery after surgical reimplantation. J Thorac Cardiovasc Surg 2021;162(4):1191–9.

50. Hernandez-Pampaloni M, Allada V, Fishbein MC, et al. Myocardial perfusion and viability by positron emission tomography in infants and children with coronary abnormalities: correlation with echocardiography, coronary angiography, and histopathology. J Am Coll Cardiol 2003;41(4):618–26.

51. Greenwood JP, Maredia N, Younger JF, et al. Cardiovascular magnetic resonance and single-photon emission computed tomography for diagnosis of coronary heart disease (CE-MARC): a prospective trial. Lancet 2012;379(9814):453–60.

52. Schwitter J, Wacker CM, Wilke N, et al. MR-IMPACT II: magnetic Resonance Imaging for Myocardial Perfusion Assessment in Coronary artery disease Trial: perfusion-cardiac magnetic resonance vs. single-photon emission computed tomography for the detection of coronary artery disease: a comparative. Eur Heart J 2013;34(10):775–81.

53. Ge Y, Antiochos P, Steel K, et al. Prognostic value of stress CMR perfusion imaging in patients with reduced left ventricular function. JACC Cardiovasc Imaging 2020. https://doi.org/10.1016/j.jcmg.2020.05.034. Published online.

54. Wahl A, Paetsch I, Gollesch A, et al. Safety and feasibility of high-dose dobutamine-atropine stress cardiovascular magnetic resonance for diagnosis of myocardial ischaemia: experience in 1000 consecutive cases. Eur Heart J 2004;25(14):1230–6.

55. Paetsch I, Jahnke C, Wahl A, et al. Comparison of dobutamine stress magnetic resonance, adenosine stress magnetic resonance, and adenosine stress magnetic resonance perfusion. Circulation 2004;110(7):835–42. doi:.FB.

56. Jahnke C, Nagel E, Gebker R, et al. Prognostic value of cardiac magnetic resonance stress tests: adenosine stress perfusion and dobutamine stress wall motion imaging. Circulation 2007;115(13):1769–76.

57. Gebker R, Jahnke C, Manka R, et al. Additional value of myocardial perfusion imaging during dobutamine stress magnetic resonance for the assessment of coronary artery disease. Circ Cardiovasc Imaging 2008;1(2):122–30.

58. Charoenpanichkit C, Hundley WG. The 20 year evolution of dobutamine stress cardiovascular magnetic resonance. J Cardiovasc Magn Reson 2010;12(1):59.

59. Nagel E, Lehmkuhl HB, Bocksch W, et al. Noninvasive diagnosis of ischemia-induced wall motion abnormalities with the use of high-dose dobutamine stress MRI: comparison with dobutamine stress echocardiography. Circulation 1999;99(6):763–70.

60. Leong-Poi H, Rim S-J, Le DE, et al. Perfusion versus function: the ischemic cascade in demand ischemia: implications of single-vessel versus multivessel stenosis. Circulation 2002;105(8):987–92.

61. Hauser M, Bengel FM, Kühn A, et al. Myocardial blood flow and flow reserve after coronary reimplantation in patients after arterial switch and Ross operation. Circulation 2001;103(14):1875–80.

62. Hauser M, Kuehn A, Hess J. Myocardial perfusion in patients with transposition of the great arteries after arterial switch operation. Circulation 2003; 107(18):2001.

63. Secinaro A, Ntsinjana H, Tann O, et al. Cardiovascular magnetic resonance findings in repaired anomalous left coronary artery to pulmonary artery connection (ALCAPA). J Cardiovasc Magn Reson 2011;13(1):1–6.

64. Prakash A, Powell AJ, Krishnamurthy R, et al. Magnetic resonance imaging evaluation of myocardial perfusion and viability in congenital and acquired pediatric heart disease. Am J Cardiol 2004;93(5): 657–61.

65. Noel C. Cardiac stress MRI evaluation of anomalous aortic origin of a coronary artery. Congenit Heart Dis 2017;12(5):627–9.

66. Pennell DJ, Sechtem UP, Higgins CB, et al. Clinical indications for cardiovascular magnetic resonance (CMR): consensus Panel report. Eur Heart J 2004;25(21):1940–65.

67. Paetsch I, Jahnke C, Fleck E, et al. Current clinical applications of stress wall motion analysis with cardiac magnetic resonance imaging. Eur J Echocardiogr 2005;6(5):317–26.

68. Wilkinson JC, Doan TT, Loar RW, et al. Myocardial stress perfusion MRI using regadenoson: a weight-based approach in infants and young children. Radiol Cardiothorac Imaging 2019;1(4): e190061.

69. Doan TT, Wilkinson JC, Loar RW, et al. Regadenoson stress perfusion cardiac magnetic resonance imaging in children with Kawasaki disease and coronary artery disease. Am J Cardiol 2019; 124(7):1125–32.

70. Strigl S, Beroukhim R, Valente AM, et al. Feasibility of dobutamine stress cardiovascular magnetic resonance imaging in children. J Magn Reson Imaging 2009;29(2):313–9.

71. Scannell CM, Hasaneen H, Greil G, et al. Automated quantitative stress perfusion cardiac magnetic resonance in pediatric patients. Front Pediatr 2021;9:1–8.

72. Agrawal H, Wilkinson JC, Noel CV, et al. Impaired myocardial perfusion on stress CMR correlates with invasive FFR in children with coronary anomalies. J Invasive Cardiol 2021;33(1):E45–51. Available at: http://www.ncbi.nlm.nih.gov/pubmed/ 33385986.

73. Doan TT, Qureshi AM, Sachdeva S, et al. Beta-blockade in intraseptal anomalous coronary artery with reversible myocardial ischemia. World J Pediatr Congenit Hear Surg 2021;12(1):145–8.

74. Doan TT, Molossi S, Qureshi AM, et al. Intraseptal anomalous coronary artery with myocardial infarction: Novel surgical approach. Ann Thorac Surg 2020;110(4):e271–4.

75. Doan TT, Zea-Vera R, Agrawal H, et al. Myocardial ischemia in children with anomalous aortic origin of a coronary artery with intraseptal course. Circ Cardiovasc Interv 2020;13(3):e008375.

76. Agrawal H, Molossi S, Alam M, et al. Anomalous coronary arteries and myocardial bridges: risk stratification in children using Novel cardiac catheterization techniques. Pediatr Cardiol 2017;38(3): 624–30.

77. Bigler MR, Ashraf A, Seiler C, et al. Hemodynamic relevance of anomalous coronary arteries originating from the opposite sinus of Valsalva-in search of the evidence. Front Cardiovasc Med 2021;7. https://doi.org/10.3389/fcvm.2020.591326.

78. Doan TT, Wilkinson JC, Agrawal H, et al. Instantaneous wave-free ratio (iFR) correlates with fractional flow reserve (FFR) assessment of coronary artery stenoses and myocardial bridges in children. J Invasive Cardiol 2020;32(5):176–9. Available at: http://www.ncbi.nlm.nih.gov/pubmed/ 32357130.

79. Vatner SF, McRitchie RJ, Braunwald E. Effects of dobutamine on left ventricular performance, coronary dynamics, and distribution of cardiac output in conscious dogs. J Clin Invest 1974;53(5):1265–73.

80. Asrress KN, Schuster A, Ali NF, et al. Myocardial haemodynamic responses to dobutamine stress compared to physiological exercise during cardiac magnetic resonance imaging. J Cardiovasc Magn Reson 2013;15(S1):15–6.

81. Bartunek J, Wijns W, Heyndrickx GR, et al. Effects of dobutamine on coronary stenosis physiology and morphology: comparison with intracoronary adenosine. Circulation 1999;100(3):243–9.

82. Escaned J, Cortés J, Flores A, et al. Importance of diastolic fractional flow reserve and dobutamine challenge in physiologic assessment of myocardial bridging. J Am Coll Cardiol 2003;42(2): 226–33.

83. Sen S, Escaned J, Malik IS, et al. Development and Validation of a new adenosine-independent index of stenosis severity from coronary wave–intensity analysis. J Am Coll Cardiol 2012;59(15): 1392–402.

84. Davies JE, Sen S, Dehbi H-M, et al. Use of the instantaneous wave-free ratio or fractional flow reserve in PCI. N Engl J Med 2017;376(19):1824–34.

85. Petraco R, van de Hoef TP, Nijjer S, et al. Baseline instantaneous wave-free ratio as a pressure-only estimation of Underlying coronary flow reserve. Circ Cardiovasc Interv 2014;7(4):492–502.

86. Götberg M, Christiansen EH, Gudmundsdottir IJ, et al. Instantaneous wave-free ratio versus fractional flow reserve to guide PCI. N Engl J Med 2017;376(19):1813–23.

87. Doan TT, Qureshi AM, Gowda S, et al. Abstract 11876: instantaneous wave-free ratio and fractional flow reserve are helpful in the assessment of anomalous aortic origin of a coronary artery. Circulation 2021;144(Suppl＼_1):A11876Z.

88. Joanna G, Ann ML, Rukmini K, et al. Physiological evaluation of anomalous aortic origin of coronary arteries and myocardial bridges. J Am Coll Cardiol 2021;77(18_Supplement_1):514.

89. Aleksandric SB, Djordjevic-Đikic AD, Dobric MR, et al. Functional assessment of myocardial bridging with conventional and diastolic fractional flow reserve: vasodilator versus inotropic provocation. J Am Heart Assoc 2021;10(13). https://doi.org/10.1161/JAHA.120.020597.

90. Angelini P, Uribe C, Monge J, et al. Origin of the right coronary artery from the opposite sinus of Valsalva in adults: characterization by intravascular ultrasonography at baseline and after stent angioplasty. Catheter Cardiovasc Interv 2015;86(2):199–208.

91. Angelini P, Velasco JA, Ott D, et al. Anomalous coronary artery arising from the opposite sinus: descriptive features and pathophysiologic mechanisms, as documented by intravascular ultrasonography. J Invasive Cardiol 2003;15(9):507–14. Available at: http://www.ncbi.nlm.nih.gov/pubmed/12947211.

92. Driesen BW, Warmerdam EG, Sieswerda G-JT, et al. Anomalous coronary artery originating from the opposite sinus of Valsalva (ACAOS), fractional flow reserve- and intravascular ultrasound-guided management in adult patients. Catheter Cardiovasc Interv 2018;92(1):68–75.

93. Heyden CM, Brock JE, Ratnayaka K, et al. Intravascular ultrasound (IVUS) provides the filling for the angiogram's crust: benefits of IVUS in pediatric interventional Cardiology. J Invasive Cardiol 2021;33(12):E978–85. Available at: http://www.ncbi.nlm.nih.gov/pubmed/34866050.

94. Stout KK, Daniels CJ, Aboulhosn JA, et al. 2018 AHA/ACC guideline for the management of adults with congenital heart disease: Executive summary: a report of the American College of Cardiology/American heart association task force on clinical practice guidelines. Circulation 2019;139(14):e637–97.

95. Brothers JA. Coronary artery anomalies in children: what is the risk? Curr Opin Pediatr 2016;28(5):590–6.

96. Jacobs ML. Anomalous aortic origin of a coronary artery: the gaps and the guidelines. J Thorac Cardiovasc Surg 2017;153(6):1462–5.

97. Martínez-Bravo LE, Mery CM. Commentary: the intercoronary pillar—not necessarily an innocent bystander. J Thorac Cardiovasc Surg 2019;158(1):218–9.

98. Mosca RS, Phoon CKL. Anomalous aortic origin of a coronary artery is not always a surgical disease. Semin Thorac Cardiovasc Surg Pediatr Card Surg Annu 2016;19(1):30–6.

99. Jegatheeswaran A, Devlin PJ, Williams WG, et al. Outcomes after anomalous aortic origin of a coronary artery repair: a Congenital Heart Surgeons' Society Study. J Thorac Cardiovasc Surg 2020;160(3):757–71.e5.

100. Law T, Dunne B, Stamp N, et al. Surgical results and outcomes after reimplantation for the management of anomalous aortic origin of the right coronary artery. Ann Thorac Surg 2016;102(1):192–8.

101. Bonilla-Ramirez C, Molossi S, Caldarone CA, et al. Anomalous aortic origin of the coronary arteries – state of the art management and surgical techniques. Semin Thorac Cardiovasc Surg Pediatr Card Surg Annu 2021;24(Im):85–94.

102. Padalino MA, Franchetti N, Hazekamp M, et al. Surgery for anomalous aortic origin of coronary arteries: a multicentre study from the European Congenital Heart Surgeons Association. Eur J Cardio-thoracic Surg 2019;56(4):696–703.

103. Yerebakan C, Ozturk M, Mota L, et al. Complete unroofing of the intramural coronary artery for anomalous aortic origin of a coronary artery: the role of commissural resuspension? J Thorac Cardiovasc Surg 2019;158(1):208–17.e2.

104. Schubert SA, Kron IL. Surgical unroofing for anomalous aortic origin of coronary arteries. Oper Tech Thorac Cardiovasc Surg 2016;21(3):162–77.

105. Sharma V, Burkhart HM, Dearani JA, et al. Surgical unroofing of anomalous aortic origin of a coronary artery: a single-center experience. Ann Thorac Surg 2014;98(3):941–5.

106. Frommelt PC, Sheridan DC, Berger S, et al. Ten-year experience with surgical unroofing of anomalous aortic origin of a coronary artery from the opposite sinus with an interarterial course. J Thorac Cardiovasc Surg 2011;142(5):1046–51.

107. Izumi K, Wilbring M, Stumpf J, et al. Direct reimplantation as an alternative approach for treatment of anomalous aortic origin of the right coronary artery. Ann Thorac Surg 2014;98(2):740–2.

108. Goda M, Meuris B, Meyns B. Right coronary translocation for anomalous origin of right coronary artery from the left coronary sinus. Interact Cardiovasc Thorac Surg 2011;13(2):201–2.

109. Jegatheeswaran A. Commentary: transection and reimplantation: Putting all your eggs in one basket? J Thorac Cardiovasc Surg 2021;162(4):1201–2.

110. Najm HK, Ahmad M. Transconal unroofing of anomalous left main coronary artery from right sinus with trans-septal course. Ann Thorac Surg 2019;108(6):e383–6.

111. Najm HK, Ahmad M, Hammoud MS, et al. Surgical Pearls of the transconal unroofing procedure - modifications and midterm outcomes. Ann Thorac Surg 2022. https://doi.org/10.1016/j.athoracsur.2022.04.027. Published online April 28.

112. Brotherton H, Philip RK. Anomalous left coronary artery from pulmonary artery (ALCAPA) in infants: a 5-year review in a defined birth cohort. Eur J Pediatr 2008;167(1):43–6.

113. Al-Dairy A, Rezaei Y, Pouraliakbar H, et al. Surgical repair for anomalous origin of the right coronary artery from the pulmonary artery. Korean Circ J 2017;47(1):144–7.

114. Williams IA, Gersony WM, Hellenbrand WE. Anomalous right coronary artery arising from the pulmonary artery: a report of 7 cases and a review of the literature. Am Heart J 2006;152(5):1004.e9-17.

115. Rajbanshi BG, Burkhart HM, Schaff HV, et al. Surgical strategies for anomalous origin of coronary artery from pulmonary artery in adults. J Thorac Cardiovasc Surg 2014;148(1):220–4.

116. Doan TT, Khan A, Lantin-Hermoso MR. Is it Just a murmur? Part 1-3. 2019. Available at: https://www.acc.org/education-and-meetings/patient-case-quizzes/2019/09/12/13/29/is-it-just-a-murmur-part-1.

117. Bland EF, White PD, Garland J. Congenital anomalies of the coronary arteries: report of an unusual case associated with cardiac hypertrophy. Am Heart J 1933;8(6):787–801.

118. Wesselhoeft H, Fawcett JS, Johnson AL. Anomalous origin of the left coronary artery from the pulmonary trunk. Its clinical spectrum, pathology, and pathophysiology, based on a review of 140 cases with seven further cases. Circulation 1968;38(2):403–25.

119. Roberts WC, Robinowitz M. Anomalous origin of the left anterior descending coronary artery from the pulmonary trunk with origin of the right and left circumflex coronary arteries from the aorta. Am J Cardiol 1984;54(10):1381–3.

120. Roberts WC. Major anomalies of coronary arterial origin seen in adulthood. Am Heart J 1986;111(5):941–63.

121. Lerberg DB, Ogden JA, Zuberbuhler JR, et al. Anomalous origin of the right coronary artery from the pulmonary artery. Ann Thorac Surg 1979;27(1):87–94.

122. Kudumula V, Mehta C, Stumper O, et al. Twenty-year outcome of anomalous origin of left coronary artery from pulmonary artery: management of mitral regurgitation. Ann Thorac Surg 2014;97(3):938–44.

123. Birk E, Stamler A, Katz J, et al. Anomalous origin of the left coronary artery from the pulmonary artery: diagnosis and postoperative follow up. Isr Med Assoc J 2000;2(2):111–4. http://www.ncbi.nlm.nih.gov/pubmed/10804930.

124. Ojala T, Salminen J, Happonen J-M, et al. Excellent functional result in children after correction of anomalous origin of left coronary artery from the pulmonary artery–a population-based complete follow-up study. Interact Cardiovasc Thorac Surg 2010;10(1):70–5.

125. Kühn A, Kasnar-Samprec J, Schreiber C, et al. Anomalous origin of the right coronary artery from the pulmonary artery (ARCAPA). Int J Cardiol 2010;139(2):e27–8.

126. Winner MW, Raman SV, Sun BC, et al. Preoperative assessment of anomalous right coronary artery arising from the main pulmonary artery. Case Rep Med 2011;2011:642126.

127. Yu Y, Wang Q-S, Wang X-F, et al. Diagnostic value of echocardiography on detecting the various types of anomalous origin of the left coronary artery from the pulmonary artery. J Thorac Dis 2020;12(3):319–28.

128. Patel SG, Frommelt MA, Frommelt PC, et al. Echocardiographic diagnosis, surgical treatment, and outcomes of anomalous left coronary artery from the pulmonary artery. J Am Soc Echocardiogr 2017;30(9):896–903.

129. Hoffman JIE. Electrocardiogram of anomalous left coronary artery from the pulmonary artery in infants. Pediatr Cardiol 2013;34(3):489–91.

130. Kouchoukos NT, Blackstone EH, Hanley FL, et al. Chapter 46 - congenital anomalies of the coronary arteries. Kirklin/Barrat-Boyes Card Surg 2012;588–97. https://doi.org/10.1016/B978-0-7020-6929-1.00058-7.

131. Takeuchi S, Imamura H, Katsumoto K, et al. New surgical method for repair of anomalous left coronary artery from pulmonary artery. J Thorac Cardiovasc Surg 1979;78(1):7–11. Available at: http://www.ncbi.nlm.nih.gov/pubmed/449387.

132. Bunton R, Jonas RA, Lang P, et al. Anomalous origin of left coronary artery from pulmonary artery. Ligation versus establishment of a two coronary artery system. J Thorac Cardiovasc Surg 1987;93(1):103–8. Available at: http://www.ncbi.nlm.nih.gov/pubmed/3796022.

133. Isomatsu Y, Imai Y, Shin'oka T, et al. Surgical intervention for anomalous origin of the left coronary artery from the pulmonary artery: the Tokyo experience. J Thorac Cardiovasc Surg 2001;121(4):792–7.

134. Jin Z, Berger F, Uhlemann F, et al. Improvement in left ventricular dysfunction after aortic reimplantation in 11 consecutive paediatric patients with anomalous origin of the left coronary artery from the pulmonary artery. Early results of a serial echocardiographic follow-up. Eur Heart J 1994;15(8):1044–9.

135. Alexi-Meskishvili V, Hetzer R, Weng Y, et al. Anomalous origin of the left coronary artery from the pulmonary artery. Early results with direct aortic reimplantation. J Thorac Cardiovasc Surg

1994;108(2):354–62. Available at: http://www.ncbi.nlm.nih.gov/pubmed/8041183.

136. Cochrane AD, Coleman DM, Davis AM, et al. Excellent long-term functional outcome after an operation for anomalous left coronary artery from the pulmonary artery. J Thorac Cardiovasc Surg 1999;117(2):332–42.

137. Vouhé PR, Tamisier D, Sidi D, et al. Anomalous left coronary artery from the pulmonary artery: results of isolated aortic reimplantation. Ann Thorac Surg 1992;54(4):621–6. ; discussion 627.

138. Cabrera AG, Chen DW, Pignatelli RH, et al. Outcomes of anomalous left coronary artery from pulmonary artery repair: beyond normal function. Ann Thorac Surg 2015;99(4):1342–7.

139. Qasim A, Doan TT, Pham TDN, et al. Poster: exercise stress testing in risk stratification of anomalous aortic origin of a coronary artery. In: Pediatric Reseacrh Symposium at Texas Children's Hospital. 2021. Available at: https://www.texaschildrens.org/sites/default/files/uploads/documents/symposia/2021/posters/90.pdf 2021.

Echocardiographic Evaluation of Successful Mitral Valve Repair or Need for a Second Pump Run in the Operating Room

Mitsuhiko Ota, MD[a],*, Takeshi Kitai, MD, PhD[b]

KEYWORDS

- Mitral regurgitation • Mitral valve repair • Intraoperative transesophageal echocardiography

---

KEY POINTS

- Intraoperative transesophageal echocardiography provides immediate diagnostic feedback and assessment of results during valve repair procedures and has become an essential guiding tool for decision-making among surgeons.
- Systematic echocardiographic evaluation of mitral valve repair based on a specific algorithm is mandatory.
- Three-dimensional transesophageal echocardiography plays a pivotal role in both preprocedural and postprocedural assessments in mitral valve repair.

INTRODUCTION

Mitral valve (MV) repair has become the gold standard surgical procedure for significant mitral regurgitation (MR).[1] The objectives of MV repair are to preserve or restore full leaflet motion, to create a good surface for leaflet coaptation, and to remodel and stabilize the entire annulus.

Detailed preoperative echocardiographic assessment of the MV apparatus is crucial for surgical planning.[2] Three-dimensional (3D) transesophageal echocardiography (TEE) plays a pivotal role in both preprocedural and postprocedural assessments in MV repair and has become widely adopted in echocardiographic laboratories and operating rooms worldwide.[3–6] In the operating room, intraoperative TEE evaluation requires accurate analysis of the MV anatomy and details of affected valve lesions.[7] Furthermore, as surgeons must rapidly decide whether cardiopulmonary bypass (CPB) should be continued to be weaning off or a second pump run should be selected, the echocardiographer conducting intraoperative TEE is required to be trained according to a certain algorithm. In particular, when the saline test results are difficult to judge the extent of residual regurgitation, evaluation by intraoperative TEE may be faster and more accurate under physiologic cardiac movement after weaning off the CPB.

The present review aimed to examine the current clinical role of intraoperative TEE in MV repair in the operating room.

This article originally appeared in *Cardiology Clinics*, Volume 39 Issue 2, May 2021.
Funding sources: None.
Declarations of interest: None.
[a] Department of Cardiovascular Center, Toranomon Hospital, 2-2-2 Toranomon, Minato-ku, Tokyo 105-8470, Japan; [b] Department of Cardiovascular Medicine, Kobe City Medical Center General Hospital, 2-1-1 Minatojima Minamimachi, Chuo-ku, Kobe 650-0047, Japan
* Corresponding author.
E-mail address: mohta5288923@gmail.com

ROLE OF INTRAOPERATIVE TRANSESOPHAGEAL ECHOCARDIOGRAPHY IN MITRAL VALVE REPAIR: WHAT IS SUCCESSFUL MITRAL VALVE REPAIR?

Echocardiographic imaging of the MV before and immediately after repair is crucial for immediate and long-term outcomes.[8–10] Postrepair echocardiographic imaging reveals the new baseline anatomy, assesses the function, and determines whether further intervention is required.

Successful MV repair is defined as a decrease in MR severity to mild or less without mitral stenosis or left ventricular outflow tract obstruction owing to systolic anterior motion (SAM). The surgeon should achieve complete MR elimination while minimizing valve area reduction.[11] An inadequate technique may result in either residual MR or mitral stenosis, which can be shown using intraoperative TEE. Such information will improve treatment options, enhance the timing of invasive therapies, and lead to advancements in repair techniques, thereby yielding better outcomes.

Quantitatively, an ideal MV repair should restore competency (MR <1+), ensure adequate patency (mean gradient of ≤ 6 mm Hg and MV area of ≤ 1.5 cm^2), and have durability (>10 years without significant MR and/or reoperation).[12–16] Because intraoperative TEE provides immediate diagnostic feedback and assessment of results during valve repair procedures, it has become an essential guiding tool for decision-making among surgeons.[11]

In the operating room, optimizing the communication between the surgeon and the cardiologist performing echocardiography is mandatory to ensure the best possible outcomes for patients. Because postprocedural echocardiographic evaluation can be conducted immediately after aortic cross-clamp release, the cardiologist must be on standby in the operating room before the completion of left atrial suture. Furthermore, obtaining information from the surgeon on how valve repair was performed is important. An online environment in which the surgical field can be viewed from all medical record terminals in the hospital enables cardiologists to observe directly the repaired valve remotely from an echocardiographic laboratory (Fig. 1). The key to successful MV repair is that the final 3D images of the repaired valve can be shared simultaneously between surgeons and cardiologist when the CPB was weaned off.

Because the procedures used in MV repair differ depending on the facility and surgeon, it

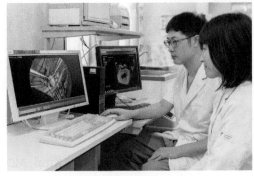

Fig. 1. Electronic medical records system that enables viewing of real-time surgical field in an echocardiographic laboratory, allowing efficient real-time information sharing between surgeons and echocardiographers.

is necessary to share information among echocardiographers on surgical techniques that are often used in daily clinical practice.

Systematic echocardiographic evaluation of MV repair is mandatory. At the initial time when the CPB is weaned off, the most sufficient imaging view for the evaluation of the repaired MV is the midesophageal (ME) long axis (LAX) view, not the 4-chamber view or mitral commissural view. The reasons for this are as follows: (1) it is easy to observe the dynamic state of the aortic valve starting to open, because the volume is loaded to the left ventricle. (2) Both the anterior and posterior MV leaflets can be visualized simultaneously. (3) The mobility, coaptation, and regurgitation of the repaired MV, as well as the iatrogenic regurgitation of the aortic valve, can be evaluated at a glance. The following checkpoints for the assessment of MV repair are recommended (Fig. 2).

Checkpoint 1: Residual Mitral Regurgitation

A successfully repaired MV should not have more than mild MR immediately after separation from the CPB.[17,18] The principles for the echocardiographic assessment of residual MR are the same as those for the evaluation of the native valve.[13] Such assessment should be performed with a sufficiently loaded left ventricle and a systolic blood pressure of greater than 100 mm Hg to simulate physiologic status and avoid residual MR underestimation. Surgeons need to put up a few minutes for proper volume and afterload settings and for their echocardiographic assessments, which results in the best benefit to patients. MR jet area with color flow Doppler (CFD) is the most common method used for the rapid quantitative evaluation of residual MR.

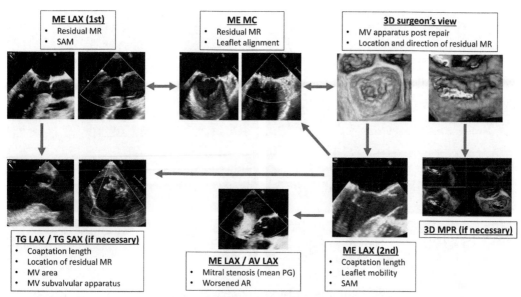

Fig. 2. Proposed TEE imaging strategy starting from the ME LAX view for MV repair. AR, aortic regurgitation; LAX, long axis; MC, mitral commissural; MPR, multiplanar reconstruction; SAX, short axis; TG, transgastric.

If residual MR is more than mild or occurs in eccentric jets, a detailed assessment is required to determine the mechanism of residual MR and aid in the revision of re-repair on a second CPB pump run (second pump run) (Fig. 3). The need for a second pump run is considered when the MR jet area is more than 1.0 cm^2 or an eccentric MR jet is observed in the authors' institution.[18]

If the site and mechanism of regurgitation cannot be evaluated accurately, the surgeon may face a problem in deciding where and how to repair the second pump run. In particular, depicting the coaptation zone of the MV in the ME LAX view is sometimes difficult owing to the acoustic shadowing caused by the annuloplasty ring implanted into the annulus. When the acceleration flow by CFD cannot be detected on the ventricular side of the repaired MV and only the regurgitant jet spreading into the left atrium can be observed, transgastric (TG) LAX and short axis views should be attempted (Fig. 4). The coaptation zone of the MV and subvalvular structures can often be clearly visualized in TG views; therefore, the detection of the acceleration flow becomes easier.

Checkpoint 2: Leaflet Mobility and Alignment

It is necessary to simultaneously observe leaflet mobility and state of coaptation while searching

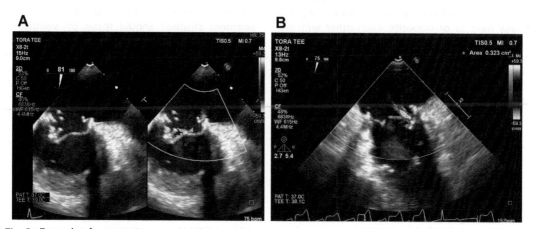

Fig. 3. Example of postrepair eccentric MR jets owing to incomplete repair. (A) Midesophageal (ME) commissural view showing eccentric MR toward the prosthetic ring caused by residual P3 prolapse. (B) ME commissural view showing eccentric MR caused by residual P1 prolapse.

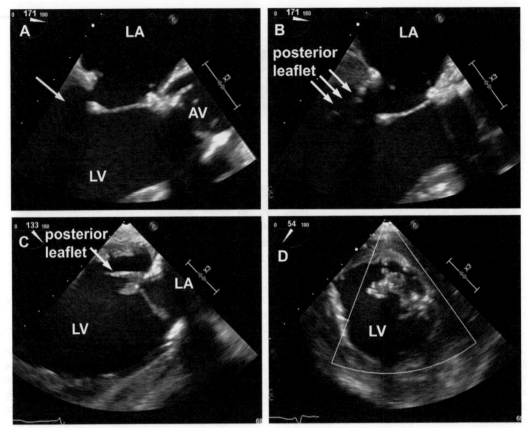

Fig. 4. Intraoperative ME TEE and TG TEE views of a case of MV repair. ME LAX views showing the repaired MV at the A2 to P2 level in peak systole (*A*) and diastole (*B*). The posterior leaflet (*arrow*) is sometimes difficult to visualize because of shadowing from the prosthetic ring (*yellow arrow*). TG LAX view of the MV at the A2 to P2 level in systole (*C*), which clearly shows the coaptation surface of the MV. The acceleration flow of residual MR can be observed with CFD in the TG short axis view of the MV at the orifice level (*D*).

for regurgitation using CFD. The ME LAX view and mitral commissural view by clockwise and counterclockwise probe rotation are applied for the assessment of leaflet appearance and motion. The leaflets' height should be aligned neatly next to or opposite each other with no coaptation gaps in systole. Additionally, an assessment of the degree and level of coaptation is essential; a successfully repaired MV should have a leaflet coaptation length of 5 to 8 mm at the A2 to P2 level (Fig. 5).[19]

Checkpoint 3: Systolic Anterior Motion

SAM refers to the dynamic movement of the MV toward the interventricular septum during systole, resulting in left ventricular outflow tract obstruction and/or MR. Because postrepair SAM is well-known to occur in 1% to 16% of patients undergoing MV repair,[20–23] the presence of SAM immediately after repair must therefore be excluded in the ME LAX view. Excessive anterior or posterior leaflet tissues, a small and

hyperkinetic left ventricle, bulging of the basal interventricular septum, and the use of a small annuloplasty ring have been identified as risk factors for SAM.[24–26] When SAM is observed during weaning from the CPB, the initial management strategy should focus on ventricular volume loading, discontinuation of inotropes, use of beta-blockers, and increasing the afterload.[27] The effects of these treatments can be observed immediately in the same ME LAX view. If significant SAM is persistent despite these medical treatments, further surgical revision is required, including reduction of the posterior leaflet's height, shortening of the neo-chords, and the use of a larger annuloplasty ring or band (Fig. 6).

When assessing the presence of SAM, it is important to ensure that all left ventricular segments begin to contract normally. Air embolism in the right coronary artery is a common complication immediately after CPB, which can lead to left ventricular inferior and posterior wall

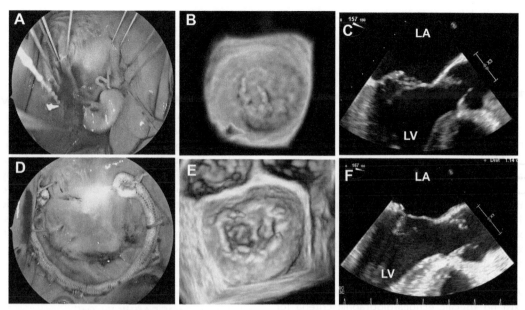

Fig. 5. A successful case of MV repair for P2 prolapse. Representative images of the MV before (*upper row; A–C*) and after (*lower row; D–F*) repair for severe MR owing to P2 prolapse. (*A*) Endoscopic view of the MV with P2 prolapse and torn chordae after placing sutures within the annulus. (*B*) A 3D photorealistic TEE surgeon's view ("True-Vue") showing a frail P2 segment and ruptured chordae tendineae. (*C*) Preoperative 2D ME LAX view showing a P2 prolapse with torn chordae. (*D*) Endoscopic view of the MV after repair during the saline test. (*E*) Intraoperative 3D TEE surgeon's view of the MV after repair at the time when the CPB was weaned off. (*F*) Postoperative 2D ME LAX view showing the coaptation surface at the A2 to P2 level.

hypokinesis with ST-segment elevation in inferior the electrocardiographic leads (II, III, and aVF). Transient abnormalities in inferior or posterior wall motion decrease the function of papillary muscles and the mobility of the mitral posterior leaflet, thereby masking the presence of SAM. Left ventricular dyssynchrony is another component that may mask postrepair SAM. Temporary epicardial pacing is routinely used to facilitate weaning from the CPB. In several cases, TEE under pacing (often around 80–90 ppm) is forced to be continued owing to the difficulty in achieving adequate sinus rhythm and sudden atrioventricular block immediately after termination from the CPB. Nonetheless, cardiac contraction often shows a nonphysiologic pattern during ventricular pacing. Furthermore, there are cases in which delayed posterolateral wall contraction is generated and the posterior leaflet does not sufficiently move during systole

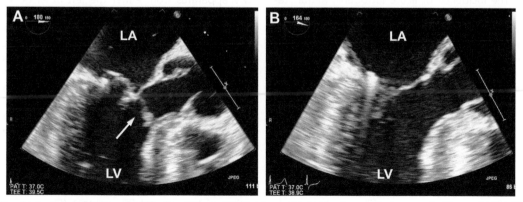

Fig. 6. An example case of SAM after MV repair requiring a second pump run and re-repair. Zoomed ME LAX views of the MV showing postrepair SAM (*arrow*) owing to excessive posterior leaflet tissue (*left, A*) and post-re-repair with shortening of the neochords after the second pump run (*right, B*).

owing to left ventricular dyssynchrony. In such cases, a significant SAM may occur as soon as an effective sinus rhythm is established. Hence, careful assessment with TEE is required because SAM may be masked when temporary cardiac pacing is indicated or the left ventricular wall motion is abnormal.

Checkpoint 4: Mitral Stenosis

The evaluation of the transvalvular flow across the MV immediately after surgery is important. Iatrogenic mitral stenosis is a recognized complication after MV repair.[28,29] Irrespective of technique, prosthetic ring or band annuloplasty is the mainstay of all repair procedures.[30] Rings or bands are used to improve the durability of repair and prevent further annular dilatation by decreasing the anatomic MV area; therefore, some degree of mitral stenosis will occur after MV repair with annuloplasty.[12,31] However, there exist no specific echocardiographic criteria for the intraoperative diagnosis of iatrogenic mitral stenosis after MV repair. Functional mitral stenosis is currently defined as an MV area of 1.5 cm^2 or less or a mean transmitral pressure gradient of 5 mm Hg or greater, irrespective of etiology. Although measurement of the anatomic MV area using 2-dimensional (2D) planimetry in the TG short axis view is useful for experienced echocardiologists, it is rarely conducted owing to technical challenges, especially in the intraoperative setting. Moreover, it is difficult to determine whether the TG short axis view is obtained at the tip level of the repaired MV and represents the smallest MV orifice area.[32] Consequently, most cardiologists and surgeons tend to rely on the mean transmitral pressure gradient to assess functional mitral stenosis after repair; nevertheless, hemodynamic changes immediately after the CPB affect this parameter.

The incidence of acute iatrogenic mitral stenosis during surgery remains unclear because the available parameters for MV area quantification in the setting immediately after repair have a different physiology, as compared with native valves. Postrepair acute mitral stenosis is rare, unless a ring that is, too small or an edge-to-edge procedure is used in multiple locations of the degenerative MV.

Checkpoint 5: Worsened Aortic Regurgitation

Postrepair TEE examination may show the emergence of a new aortic regurgitation or deterioration in preexisting aortic insufficiency if the aortic valve is injured or distorted during MV and/or tricuspid valve repair or replacement.[33–35] This iatrogenic injury to the aortic valve results from its anatomic proximity to the mitral annulus and annuloplasty ring stitches. The anterior mitral annulus is closely related to the aortic valve, specifically to the left and noncoronary aortic cusps. Normally, the distance between the nadir of these cusps and the anterior MV annulus is 5 to 10 mm; however, anatomic variations in the position of the nadir of the aortic valve and unintentional stitches may occur, resulting in suture needle perforation of the aortic cusp. Furthermore, tension caused by the MV annuloplasty ring or tricuspid valve replacement may lead to distortion of the aortic annulus owing to its adjacent position.[36] Thus, close attention should be paid to the emergence of a new aortic regurgitation after MV repair.

THE ROLE OF 3-DIMENSIONAL TRANSESOPHAGEAL ECHOCARDIOGRAPHY IN THE ASSESSMENT OF MITRAL VALVE REPAIR

Multiplane imaging with 2D TEE provides detailed assessment of cross-sectional valve anatomy and function. Although multiple thin 2D images can be mentally reconstructed into a 3D valve model, this process requires physicians to be skilled in acquiring 2D valve images with correct alignment of imaging planes according to a systematic imaging algorithm.[37] Real-time 3D TEE has improved and provided incremental value to the assessment of anatomic features, location, and extent of MV pathology.[38–41] Additionally, 3D TEE with CFD aids in identifying the location of the regurgitant orifice and direction of the regurgitant flow (Fig. 7). Real-time, single-beat 3D imaging is less operator dependent and enables the visualization of the entire MV in a single view as well as an assessment of the MV apparatus from either the left atrial or left ventricular perspective.[42,43] Furthermore, 3D TEE is superior to 2D TEE with respect to the identification of dominant lesions in patients with complex prolapse involving Barlow's disease and/or commissural lesions (Fig. 8).[44] The amount of commissural tissues varies greatly, and commissures sometimes exist as distinct leaflet scallops. In addition, 3D TEE is useful for recognizing the indentations that separate the posterior leaflet into 3 individual scallops.[45,46] The location of these indentations considerably varies among individuals, and there is also a bulky P3 scallop that is large enough to occupy the position of the original P2 segment (Fig. 9). This recognition is essential when planning procedures such as indentation closure in MV repair.

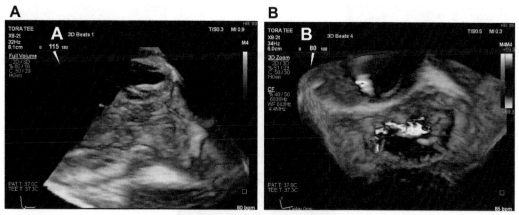

Fig. 7. Real-time 3D TG LAX view can easily shows the coaptation zone of the MV with only a single-beat acquisition (*A*). 3D multi-beat CFD of repaired MV can demonstrates an eccentric jet from P3 segment (*B*).

Acquisition of 3D datasets is mandatory, which is ideal when assessing complex structures of the MV apparatus in detail. Multibeat, wide angle, full-volume 3D imaging can provide images with greater temporal and spatial resolution.[3,45] Nonetheless, multibeat 3D imaging requires electrocardiographic-gated acquisition and breath holds to minimize stitch artifacts, and it takes considerable experience for echocardiographers to capture high-quality 3D TEE images without artifacts.

Performing TEE for detailed preoperative evaluation in the operating room is not recommended because electrocautery-induced electrical interference has a negative effect on electrocardiographic-gated images and echocardiographic image quality is likely to be poor owing to the patients' supine position instead of left lateral position.

Surgeons have ethical duties to explain planned procedures to patients and obtain valid informed consent from patients before surgery. Therefore, preoperative TEE should be completed in the echocardiographic laboratory rather than in the operating room on the day of surgery. Furthermore, 3D TEE facilitates communication with surgeons by providing images that they may see upon opening up the left atrium in the operating room. Further advancements in imaging will continue to improve the understanding about

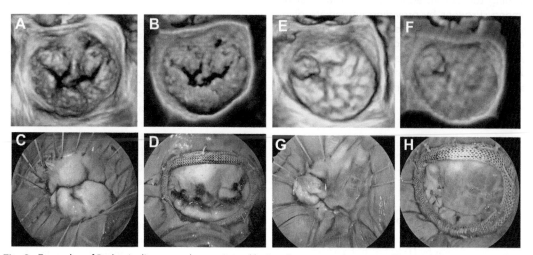

Fig. 8. Examples of Barlow's disease and commissural lesion. Representative cases of severe MR owing to Barlow's disease (*A–D*) and commissural lesion (*E–H*) are shown in 3D TEE images and endoscopic views before and after repair. Preoperative 3D surgeon's view from the left atrial perspective (*A, E*). Photorealistic 3D surgeon's view (*B, F*). Preoperative endoscopic view (*C, G*). Postoperative endoscopic view immediately after repair during the saline test (*D, H*).

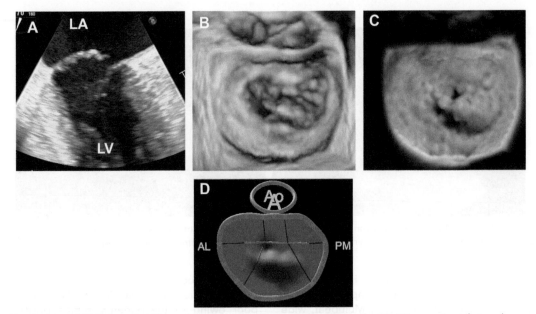

Fig. 9. A bulky P3 lesion mimicking a P2 lesion in conventional 2D images. The 2D ME commissural view shows a huge P3 lesion that is about to reach the P1 segment over the original P2 segment (*A*). These 3D surgeon's views are more intuitive for understanding the anatomic characteristics and mechanism of regurgitation (*B*). A 3D photo-realistic view ("TrueVue") provides additional anatomic details (*C*). Peak systolic parametric map derived from a 3D TEE image showing prolapse of the huge P3 scallop over the P2 scallop area (*D*).

MV function and dysfunction both before and after repair.

SUMMARY

TEE is an important preoperative imaging modality for successful MV repair and an essential guiding tool for intraoperative decision-making among surgeons by providing immediate diagnostic feedback and assessment of results during valve repair procedures. Systematic echocardiographic evaluation of MV repair and use of 3D TEE in combination with 2D TEE based on a specific algorithm are mandatory.

CLINICS CARE POINTS

- Successful mitral valve (MV) repair is defined as a decrease in mitral regurgitation (MR) severity to mild or less without mitral stenosis (MS) or systolic anterior motion (SAM).

- Intraoperative transesophageal echocardiography (TEE) has become an essential guiding tool for decision-making among surgeons.

- Systematic echocardiographic evaluation according to the following checkpoints,

including residual MR, leaflet mobility and alignment, SAM, iatrogenic MS, and worsened aortic regurgitation should be performed immediately after MV repair.

REFERENCES

1. David TE, Armstrong S, McCrindle BW, et al. Late outcomes of mitral valve repair for mitral regurgitation due to degenerative disease. Circulation 2013; 127:1485–92.

2. Nishimura RA, Otto CM, Bonow RO, et al. Thomas JD and American College of Cardiology/American Heart Association Task Force on practice G. 2014 AHA/ACC guideline for the management of patients with valvular heart disease: executive summary: a report of the American College of Cardiology/American Heart Association Task Force on practice guidelines. J Am Coll Cardiol 2014;63: 2438–88.

3. Nicoara A, Skubas N, Ad N, et al. Guidelines for the use of transesophageal echocardiography to assist with surgical decision-making in the operating room: a surgery-based approach: from the American Society of Echocardiography in Collaboration with the Society of Cardiovascular Anesthesiologists and the Society of Thoracic Surgeons. J Am Soc Echocardiogr 2020;33:692–734.

4. La Canna G, Arendar I, Maisano F, et al. Real-time three-dimensional transesophageal echocardiography for assessment of mitral valve functional anatomy in patients with prolapse-related regurgitation. Am J Cardiol 2011;107:1365–74.

5. Ahmed S, Nanda NC, Miller AP, et al. Usefulness of transesophageal three-dimensional echocardiography in the identification of individual segment/scallop prolapse of the mitral valve. Echocardiography 2003;20:203–9.

6. Ben Zekry S, Nagueh SF, Little SH, et al. Comparative accuracy of two- and three-dimensional transthoracic and transesophageal echocardiography in identifying mitral valve pathology in patients undergoing mitral valve repair: initial observations. J Am Soc Echocardiogr 2011;24:1079–85.

7. Mahmood F, Matyal R. A quantitative approach to the intraoperative echocardiographic assessment of the mitral valve for repair. Anesth Analg 2015; 121:34–58.

8. Shah PM, Raney AA, Duran CM, et al. Multiplane transesophageal echocardiography: a roadmap for mitral valve repair. J Heart Valve Dis 1999;8: 625–9.

9. Sidebotham DA, Allen SJ, Gerber IL, et al. Intraoperative transesophageal echocardiography for surgical repair of mitral regurgitation. J Am Soc Echocardiogr 2014;27:345–66.

10. Hahn RT, Abraham T, Adams MS, et al, American Society of E and Society of Cardiovascular A. Guidelines for performing a comprehensive transesophageal echocardiographic examination: recommendations from the American Society of Echocardiography and the Society of Cardiovascular Anesthesiologists. Anesth Analg 2014;118: 21–68.

11. Adams DH, Anyanwu AC, Sugeng L, et al. Degenerative mitral valve regurgitation: surgical echocardiography. Curr Cardiol Rep 2008;10:226–32.

12. Ibrahim MF, David TE. Mitral stenosis after mitral valve repair for non-rheumatic mitral regurgitation. Ann Thorac Surg 2002;73:34–6.

13. Zoghbi WA, Adams D, Bonow RO, et al. Recommendations for noninvasive evaluation of native valvular regurgitation: a report from the American Society of echocardiography Developed in Collaboration with the Society for Cardiovascular Magnetic Resonance. J Am Soc Echocardiogr 2017;30: 303–71.

14. Brinster DR, Unic D, D'Ambra MN, et al. Midterm results of the edge-to-edge technique for complex mitral valve repair. Ann Thorac Surg 2006; 81:1612–7.

15. Riegel AK, Busch R, Segal S, et al. Evaluation of transmitral pressure gradients in the intraoperative echocardiographic diagnosis of mitral stenosis after mitral valve repair. PLoS One 2011;6:e26559.

16. Kasegawa H, Shimokawa T, Horai T, et al. Long-term echocardiography results of mitral valve repair for mitral valve prolapse. J Heart Valve Dis 2008;17: 162–7.

17. Suri RM, Clavel MA, Schaff HV, et al. Effect of recurrent mitral regurgitation following degenerative mitral valve repair: long-term analysis of competing outcomes. J Am Coll Cardiol 2016;67:488–98.

18. Tabata M, Kasegawa H, Fukui T, et al. Long-term outcomes of artificial chordal replacement with tourniquet technique in mitral valve repair: a single-center experience of 700 cases. J Thorac Cardiovasc Surg 2014;148:2033–2038 e1.

19. Uchimuro T, Tabata M, Saito K, et al. Post-repair coaptation length and durability of mitral valve repair for posterior mitral valve prolapse. Gen Thorac Cardiovasc Surg 2014;62:221–7.

20. Ibrahim M, Rao C, Ashrafian H, et al. Modern management of systolic anterior motion of the mitral valve. Eur J Cardiothorac Surg 2012;41:1260–70.

21. Jebara VA, Mihaileanu S, Acar C, et al. Left ventricular outflow tract obstruction after mitral valve repair. Results of the sliding leaflet technique. Circulation 1993;88:II30–4.

22. Lee KS, Stewart WJ, Lever HM, et al. Mechanism of outflow tract obstruction causing failed mitral valve repair. Anterior displacement of leaflet coaptation. Circulation 1993;88:II24–9.

23. Crescenzi G, Landoni G, Zangrillo A, et al. Management and decision-making strategy for systolic anterior motion after mitral valve repair. J Thorac Cardiovasc Surg 2009;137:320–5.

24. Maslow AD, Regan MM, Haering JM, et al. Echocardiographic predictors of left ventricular outflow tract obstruction and systolic anterior motion of the mitral valve after mitral valve reconstruction for myxomatous valve disease. J Am Coll Cardiol 1999;34:2096–104.

25. Shah PM, Raney AA. Echocardiographic correlates of left ventricular outflow obstruction and systolic anterior motion following mitral valve repair. J Heart Valve Dis 2001;10:302–6.

26. Manabe S, Kasegawa H, Fukui T, et al. Morphological analysis of systolic anterior motion after mitral valve repair. Interact Cardiovasc Thorac Surg 2012;15:235–9.

27. Brown ML, Abel MD, Click RL, et al. Systolic anterior motion after mitral valve repair: is surgical intervention necessary? J Thorac Cardiovasc Surg 2007; 133:136–43.

28. Maslow A. Mitral valve repair: an echocardiographic review: part 2. J Cardiothorac Vasc Anesth 2015;29:439–71.

29. Essandoh M. Intraoperative echocardiographic assessment of mitral valve area after degenerative mitral valve repair: a call for guidelines or recommendations. J Cardiothorac Vasc Anesth 2016;30: 1364–8.

30. Bothe W, Miller DC, Doenst T. Sizing for mitral annuloplasty: where does science stop and voodoo begin? Ann Thorac Surg 2013;95:1475–83.

31. Mesana TG, Lam BK, Chan V, et al. Clinical evaluation of functional mitral stenosis after mitral valve repair for degenerative disease: potential affect on surgical strategy. J Thorac Cardiovasc Surg 2013;146:1418–23 [discussion: 1423–5].

32. Maslow A, Mahmood F, Poppas A, et al. Three-dimensional echocardiographic assessment of the repaired mitral valve. J Cardiothorac Vasc Anesth 2014;28:11–7.

33. Hill AC, Bansal RC, Razzouk AJ, et al. Echocardiographic recognition of iatrogenic aortic valve leaflet perforation. Ann Thorac Surg 1997;64:684–9.

34. Rother A, Smith B, Adams DH, et al. Transesophageal echocardiographic diagnosis of acute aortic valve insufficiency after mitral valve repair. Anesth Analg 2000;91:499–500.

35. Lakew F, Urbanski PP. Aortic valve leaflet perforation after minimally invasive mitral valve repair. Ann Thorac Surg 2016;101:1180–2.

36. Veronesi F, Caiani EG, Sugeng L, et al. Effect of mitral valve repair on mitral-aortic coupling: a real-time three-dimensional transesophageal echocardiography study. J Am Soc Echocardiogr 2012;25:524–31.

37. Poelaert JI, Bouchez S. Perioperative echocardiographic assessment of mitral valve regurgitation: a comprehensive review. Eur J Cardiothorac Surg 2016;50:801–12.

38. Tsang W, Weinert L, Sugeng L, et al. The value of three-dimensional echocardiography derived mitral valve parametric maps and the role of experience in the diagnosis of pathology. J Am Soc Echocardiogr 2011;24:860–7.

39. Chandra S, Salgo IS, Sugeng L, et al. Characterization of degenerative mitral valve disease using morphologic analysis of real-time three-dimensional echocardiographic images: objective insight into complexity and planning of mitral valve repair. Circ Cardiovasc Imaging 2011;4:24–32.

40. Drake DH, Zimmerman KG, Hepner AM, et al. Echo-guided mitral repair. Circ Cardiovasc Imaging 2014;7:132–41.

41. Maffessanti F, Marsan NA, Tamborini G, et al. Quantitative analysis of mitral valve apparatus in mitral valve prolapse before and after annuloplasty: a three-dimensional intraoperative transesophageal study. J Am Soc Echocardiogr 2011;24:405–13.

42. Grewal J, Suri R, Mankad S, et al. Mitral annular dynamics in myxomatous valve disease: new insights with real-time 3-dimensional echocardiography. Circulation 2010;121:1423–31.

43. Lang RM, Badano LP, Tsang W, et al, American Society of E and European Association of E. EAE/ASE recommendations for image acquisition and display using three-dimensional echocardiography. Eur Heart J Cardiovasc Imaging 2012;13:1–46.

44. Tsang W, Lang RM. Three-dimensional echocardiography is essential for intraoperative assessment of mitral regurgitation. Circulation 2013;128:643–52 [discussion: 652].

45. Ring L, Rana BS, Ho SY, et al. The prevalence and impact of deep clefts in the mitral leaflets in mitral valve prolapse. Eur Heart J Cardiovasc Imaging 2013;14:595–602.

46. Mantovani F, Clavel MA, Vatury O, et al. Cleft-like indentations in myxomatous mitral valves by three-dimensional echocardiographic imaging. Heart 2015;101:1111–7.

Tricuspid Regurgitation and Right Heart Failure
The Role of Imaging in Defining Pathophysiology, Presentation, and Novel Management Strategies

Vratika Agarwal, MD*, Rebecca Hahn, MD

KEYWORDS
• Tricuspid regurgitation • Right heart failure • Transcatheter tricuspid valve intervention

KEY POINTS
• Understanding the anatomy of tricuspid valve and physiology of tricuspid valve function, is integral to understanding the development of tricuspid regurgitation and the relationhip to right heart and pulmonary vascular function.
• Multimodality imaging plays a crucial role in delineating the etiology of TR, anatomy of the tricuspid valve as well as effects of TR on pulmonary vascular system and right ventricle.
• Defining the morphology and clinical etiology of TR and understanding the associated differences in outcome is paramount to both the optimization of current treatments as well as for development of new treatment options for TR.

During the last few years, there has been a substantial shift in efforts to understand and manage secondary or functional tricuspid regurgitation (TR) given its prevalence, adverse prognostic impact, and symptom burden associated with progressive right heart failure.[1] The previously "forgotten valve" has gained tremendous attention due to advances in novel treatment strategies; however, the timing and impact of intervention is not well understood. Recent study shows that the age-adjusted prevalence of TR is about 0.55% with an increasing incidence in population aged older than 75 years[2] with secondary or functional TR the most common cause.[3] Understanding the pathophysiology of TR and right heart failure is crucial for determining the best treatment strategy and improving outcomes. In this article, we review the complex relationship between right heart

structural and hemodynamic changes that drive the pathophysiology of secondary TR and discuss the role of multimodality imaging in the diagnosis, management, and determination of outcomes.

TRICUSPID VALVE AND RIGHT HEART ANATOMY

To understand the pathophysiologic relationship between right heart structure and function and mechanisms of secondary TR, it is important to appreciate the complex anatomy of the tricuspid valve (TV) and the right ventricle (RV). TV is distinct from the other valves in its anatomical variability and complexity. The TV apparatus is composed of (1) the tricuspid anulus (TA), (2) leaflets, (3) subvalvular chordae, and (4) papillary muscles.[4] The TV is the largest valve in the body,

This article originally appeared in *Heart Failure Clinics*, Volume 19 Issue 4, October 2023.
Division of Cardiology, Department of Medicine, Columbia University Medical Center/ New York Presbyterian Hospital, 177 Fort Washington Avenue, Room 5C-501, New York, NY 10032, USA
* Corresponding author. 177 Fort Washington Avenue, Room 5C-501, New York, NY 10032.
E-mail address: va2374@cumc.columbia.edu

with a saddle-shaped TA (high points at the septum and lateral wall) with a dynamic change in shape during the cardiac cycle to ensure maximum flow across the valve in diastole and achieve coaptation during systole.[5] There is very little fibrous tissue or collagen along the RV free wall segment of the TA[6] with greater cellularity and organized elastic fibers in men compared with women.[7] Normal women also have larger indexed TA dimensions and area and thus may be predisposed to developing TR. In fact, by the eighth decade of life, significant TR is 4 times more prevalent in women than in men.[8] Atrial fibrillation results in dilation of the TA and blunting of the dynamic change in TA shape, contributing to the progression of TR.[9]

The tricuspid leaflets are thin and highly variable in size and number.[10] The main support for the anterior and posterior leaflets is complex chordal arcades that originate from a large anterior papillary muscle, attached to the moderator band and lateral RV wall. A variable number of posterior papillary muscles subtend the variable number of posterior leaflets. Unique to this right atrioventricular valve are the numerous direct chordal attachments from the interventricular septum to the septal leaflet(s) and often portions of the anterior leaflet. Alteration of any of these structures may lead to malcoaptation the leaflet tips and TR.

The RV is the anterior most chamber of the heart and lies close to the chest wall and can be divided into 3 parts—the inlet, the body, and the outlet.[11,12] Muscle fibers are arranged in 2 layers with the outer myocytes arranged circumferentially and inner layer of longitudinal fibers. The RV contracts by 3 separate mechanisms[1]: movement of the free wall toward the septum, which produces a bellowing effect[2]; traction on the free wall at the points of attachment to left ventricular (LV) as well as contraction of the superficial fibres connecting the LV-RV; and contraction of the longitudinal fibers, which shortens the long axis and draws the TA toward the apex.[11] Unlike the LV, which relies on oblique muscle fibers, the majority of the RV function is driven by contraction of the longitudinal muscle fibers. However, RV systolic function is highly reliant on pulmonary pressures (afterload), preload as well as contractile function of the RV. The RV has long been thought to be more sensitive than the LV to acute increases in afterload[13] with experimental models showing that a pressure load on the RV is less well tolerated than a volume load.[14] In response to pressure overload, the RV remodeling is initially adaptive, characterized by more concentric hypertrophy with mild RV dilatation, with preserved systolic and diastolic function.[15] With progression of the primary disease process, there is maladaptive remodeling associated with more eccentric hypertrophy and thus marked RV dilatation and reduced systolic and diastolic function.[16] With RV dilatation, there is a loss of longitudinal RV function; however, recruitment of circumferential myocytes preserves RV stroke volume.

PATHOPHYSIOLOGY OF SECONDARY TRICUSPID REGURGITATION

Several studies evaluating predictors of TR severity and progression have resulted in a more comprehensive understanding of TR pathophysiology. Maladaptive RV remodeling in the setting of increased afterload (ie, pulmonary hypertension [PH]) will significantly affect TV function due to changes in the position of the papillary muscles (toward the apex), thus stretching of the tricuspid chordae leading to tenting or tethering of the leaflets, which results in leaflet malcoaptation.[17] More than mild TR is indeed predicted by end-systolic RV eccentricity index greater than 2.0 (area under the curve [AUC] 0.90), TV tethering area greater than 1.0 cm^2 (AUC 0.75), and end-diastolic TA diameter greater than 3.9 cm (AUC 0.65).[18] Recent studies however have shown that right atrial (RA) volume is a better predictor of TA area in secondary TR than RV end-diastolic volume, irrespective of cardiac rhythm and RV loading conditions.[19] This same study showed that the largest RA volume and smallest RV volumes were seen in patients with atrial fibrillation and secondary TR. Other studies confirm that atrial fibrillation is associated with larger RA volumes and TA areas in patients with TR[20] and is a predictor of TR progression along with an elevated pulmonary artery systolic pressure (PASP) of 36 mm Hg or greater.[21]

Given these clear morphologic differences, a more granular classification scheme has been developed, which not only includes differences in TV leaflet pathologic condition and mode of coaptation but also includes characteristic differences in TA, RV, and RA remodeling related to the distinct pathophysiology of secondary TR.[22,23]

CLASSIFICATION OF TRICUSPID REGURGITATION

The new classification scheme for TR challenges the simple classification of TR into primary disease defined as pathology of the leaflets, and secondary disease with intrinsically normal leaflets but abnormalities of the other TV apparatus. This classification scheme now recognizes the different morphologic entities of atrial and ventricular secondary TR, and a separate category of cardiac implantable electronic device (CIED)-related TR (Table 1).

Common causes of primary TR are shown in Fig. 1. Congenital causes of primary TR include: (1) Ebstein anomaly characterized by apical displacement of the TV leaflets, which originate from the RV with variable chordae resulting in atrialization of the RV; (2) atrioventricular canal resulting from failure of superior and inferior endocardium to fuse during embryologic development; and (3) TV dysplasia described as congenital malformation of the TV apparatus. In adults, the most common causes of primary TR include: (1) myxomatous degeneration of the TV; (2) systemic disease process including connective tissue disorders (sarcoidosis, lupus erythematosus, rheumatic disease); (3) infective endocarditis; (4) carcinogenic pathology (carcinoid, tumors involving right heart); (5) drug-induced inflammatory reaction (ergot derivatives, dopamine agonists, and anorectic medications);

(6) chest wall trauma with injury to the RV and TV; and (7) trauma (biopsy or deceleration injury).

Although CIED leads have been classically categorized as a primary cause of TR, it is the device lead that has the direct effect on the leaflets or subvalvular apparatus and, thus, is considered a separate cause of TR.[24,25] CIED-induced TR may occur due to leaflet impingement by the lead without injury to the TV apparatus, or perforation of the leaflet, or adhesions/interference with the subvalvular apparatus (Fig. 2). CIED-induced is one of the most common causes of acquired TR with incidence of TR around 38% after lead placement.[26] CIED-induced TR is associated with a mortality of 10% to 20%.[27] The presence of a CIED is a strong predictor of progression of rapid progression og TR.[28] All-cause mortality (>1 year after pacemaker implantation) was higher in patients with TR deterioration (hazard ratio, 1.598; 95% CI, 1.275–2.002; $P < .01$).[25]

Ventricular secondary TR is characterized by dilatation, often in the midventricle resulting in a more spherical RV, RV dysfunction, and tethering of the TV leaflets. This cause is seen with pulmonary arterial hypertension, left-sided valvulopathy, and LV dysfunction.[29,30] Left-sided disease commonly results in pulmonary venous

Table 1
Classification of tricuspid regurgitation

Primary Tricuspid Regurgitation	Secondary Tricuspid Regurgitation	CIED-Related Tricuspid Regurgitation
Congenital 1. Ebstein anomaly 2. Atrioventricular canal defects 3. Tricuspid valve dysplasia	Atrial functional 1. Normal LV systolic function 2. Severe atrial dilatation 3. Absence of apical tethering of TV leaflets	CIED-induced leaflet impingement
Myxomatous degeneration	Ventricular functional due to left-sided disease 4. Left ventricular systolic dysfunction 5. Aortic valve disease 6. Mitral valve disease	
Systemic disease 1. Sarcoidosis 2. Lupus erythematosus 3. Rheumatic disease	Primary Right ventricular disease: 1) Right ventricular myopathy 2) RV ischemia 3)Arrhythmogenic right ventricular cardiomyopathy	
Malignancy 1. Carcinoid 2. Tumors involving right heart	Severe primary pulmonary hypertension	
Infective Endocarditis		
Iatrogenic causes 1. RV biopsy		
Chest wall trauma		
Drug induced		

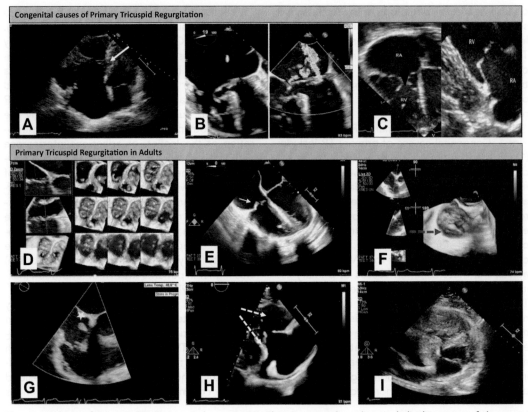

Fig. 1. Etiology of Primary TR. Congenital causes: (A) Ebstein anomaly with apical displacement of the septal leaflet (*white arrow*). (B) Atrio-ventricular canal defect. (C) Tricuspid atresia with abnormal development of the TV leaflets. Causes of Primary TR in adults (D) Prolapse: Multiplanar imaging showing short axis image of myxomatous TV with multileaflet thickening and prolapse. (E) Iatrogenic: Flail anterior leaflet (*yellow arrow*) following right heart biopsy. (F) Rheumatic disease of the TV with commissural fusion (*red dotted arrow*) (G) Endocarditis with vegetation on the atrial aspect of the anterior leaflet (*star*). (H) Carcinoid disease with thickened and fixed anterior and septal leaflets (*dotted white arrows*). (I) Angiosarcoma involving the RV.

hypertension. Both pulmonary arterial, pulmonary venous, and mixed PH result in an increase in RV afterload and the cascade of adaptive and maladaptive changes resulting in TR (Fig. 3). Ventricular secondary TR in the presence of LV dysfunction (LVEF <50%), PH (PASP >50 mm Hg), and left-sided valvular disease carries a yearly mortality approaching 30%.[2]

Atrial secondary TR is characterized by less-prominent RV dilatation and therefore less TV leaflet tethering but marked dilatation of the TA and RA (Fig. 3).[31,32] Atrial functional TR is an increasingly recognized entity more so due to heightened awareness of atrial functional mitral regurgitation and its prognostic implications.[33,34] Recent studies have attempted to clearly define the clinical and morphologic characteristics of the disease. Based on a clustering approach, Schlotter and colleagues defined atrial secondary TR as TV tenting height of 10 mm or lesser, midventricular RV diameter of

38 mm or lesser, and LV ejection fraction of 50% or greater.[35] Atrial secondary TR has a yearly mortality of only 10% to 15%.[2] In patients treated with transcatheter TV intervention (TTVI), atrial secondary TR was independently associated with a lower rate of the combined end point of mortality and heart failure hospitalization at 1-year follow-up (hazard ratio, 0.39; P<.05). Despite limited evidence to date, rhythm control may help to decrease atrial secondary TR in some patients through reverse remodeling of RA and TA.[36,37] Moreover, this form may be particularly amenable to treatment with annuloplasty devices because leaflet tethering is typically minimal.[19,38]

CLINICAL PRESENTATION

In the past, right-sided valvular disease and right heart failure have received less consideration from clinicians than left-sided disease. The

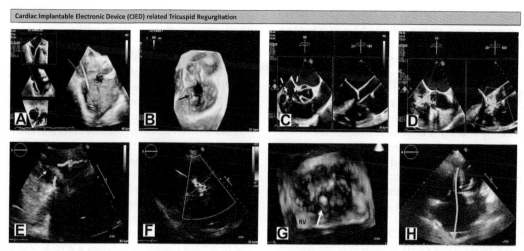

Fig. 2. CIED-related TR. (A) Septal-lateral and posterior trajectory of the pacemaker lead showing impingement of the posterior leaflet (*red arrow*). (B) Three-dimensional en face view showing pacemaker lead impingement at the level of the leaflet (*black arrow*). (C) Multiple pacemaker wires (*yellow dotted arrows*) noted crossing the TV annulus. (D) Regurgitant jets noted around both device wires. (E) Impingement of the subvalvular apparatus (*white arrow*). (F) regurgitant jet originating at the subvalvular level at the site of impingement. (G) Three-dimensional view from the RV showing subvalvular impingement (*white arrow*). (H) Septal trajectory taken by the distal end of the lead causing subvalvular impingement (*yellow arrow*).

heterogeneity of the disease process and its dependence with loading conditions, PH, hemodynamic alterations, rhythm abnormalities, co-morbid conditions, and other contributing diseases have often confused care providers regarding the optimal timing of intervention. In the recent years, the focus has shifted to early identification and treatment because several studies have demonstrated the ominous impact of significant TR on mortality and morbidity with or without concomitant left-sided disease.[39,40]

Symptoms of TR are often nonspecific and covert. Due to the long latency period of severe TR, patients are referred for treatment during

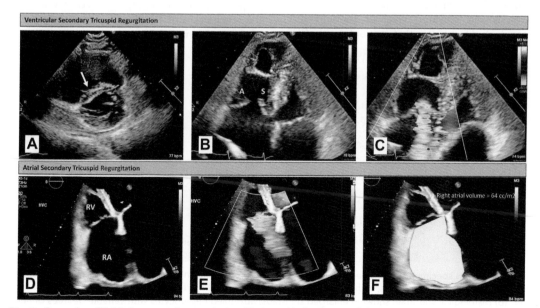

Fig. 3. Secondary TR (A) Severe right ventricular dilation with flattening of the interventricular septum (*white arrow*). (B) Apical tethering of the anterior and septal leaflet with large central coaptation gap. (C) Severe central TR. (D) Severe RA dilatation with RA larger than the RV. (E) Multiple regurgitant central jets. (F) RA volumetric assessment.

advanced stages. During the initial stages of the disease process, severe TR may be well tolerated. The symptoms with atrial functional TR in its isolated form are usually fatigue and exercise intolerance. This is due to poor cardiac output and loss of atrio-ventricular synchrony due to chronic atrial fibrillation. There is chronic elevation of RA pressure, which may result in congestive hepatopathy and signs of venous congestion.

Conversely, a long-standing TR or TR with RV remodeling is associated with overt signs of right heart failure resulting in ascites, loss of appetite, hepatic dysfunction, and anasarca. Cardiohepatic syndrome (CHS) is often noted in patients with chronic TR with persistently elevated RA pressures. CHS is mainly classified into 2 types. Type I CHS is seen in acute decompensated heart failure resulting in hypoxic or ischemic hepatitis and shock liver. This results in hepatocellular death either due to hypoperfusion and necrosis (elevated transaminases) or cholestasis due to systemic congestion (elevated bilirubin, alkaline phosphatase, and gamma glutamyl transferase). Type 2 CHS is associated with chronic heart failure and is often referred to as congestive hepatopathy. This results in sinusoidal dilatation commonly referred to as nut meg liver on histological examination (Fig. 4). Transaminases in this population are usually within the reference range with elevated levels of bilirubin, alkaline phosphatase, and gamma glutamyl transferase.[41] Biventricular failure may lead to microcirculatory dysfunction and cellular cytolysis and elevated level of transaminase. Recent study showed that patients with CHS who underwent TTVI had worse outcomes when compared with those without.[42] Degree of hepatic impairment should be an important consideration for risk stratifying patients before intervention and all efforts must be made to recognize hepatic decline at an early stage when TV intervention may lead to hepatic regeneration and restoration of function.

CHS is often accompanied by cardiorenal syndrome (CRS). CRS is the interaction of cardiac and renal function and vice-versa during an ongoing disease process. There are 5 types of CRS: types 1 and 2 reflect the impact of acute and chronic diseases of the heart, respectively, on the renal function and vice versa, the effects of acute and chronic diseases of the kidney on the heart are classified as types 3 and 4, respectively. Type 5 is concomitant impact on both organs due to a common systemic illness effecting both organs.[43] Studies have shown reduction in abdominal congestion and stable or reduction in diuretic doses after TTVI; however, improvement in renal function after intervention was not demonstrated.[44–46]

ROLE OF IMAGING IN TRICUSPID REGURGITATION

In the era of emerging new therapies for management of TV disease, multimodality imaging plays a crucial role in preprocedural, intraprocedural, and postprocedural assessments. Imaging plays a vital role in identifying and differentiating the mechanism of TR as well as the assessment of right heart function.

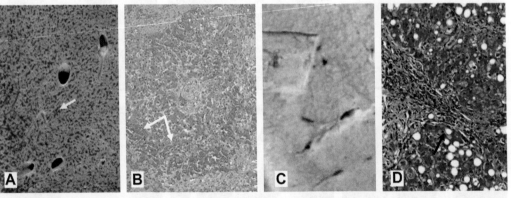

Fig. 4. (A) Gross specimen showing reddish central areas that represent sinusoidal congestion (*yellow arrow*) and bleeding in the atrophied regions, with contrasting yellowish discoloration representing either normal liver or fatty liver. (B) Histological specimen showing enlarged sinusoids, atrophied hepatocytes with variable degrees of hemorrhage (*white arrows*). (C) Gross specimen from alcoholic cirrhosis showing nodularity. Cirrhosis due to other causes often results in the loss of normal lobular architecture of hepatic parenchyma and replacement with regenerative nodules and fibrous tissue. (D) Histological specimen showing fibrous septa that divide the hepatic parenchyma into nodules (*black arrow*).

Transthoracic Echocardiography (TTE): TTE is the ideal initial imaging modality and serves to establish the diagnosis. TTE besides being an easily accessible, noninvasive modality with high temporal resolution is unique in its ability to image the TV and the right heart. Due to the proximity of the right heart to chest wall owing to the anterior position, TV is a near field structure and imaging from parasternal views provides excellent anatomical and functional evaluation.[47] The primary objectives of the echocardiogram are as follows:

1. Define TV anatomy
2. Determine the cause of TR
3. Assess the severity of TR by both qualitative and quantitative methods
4. Characterize right ventricular and RA anatomy and function
5. Assess for other associated valvular pathologic condition and left-sided function
6. Image extracardiac structures—inferior vena cava (IVC) and superior vena cava (SVC)
7. Assess flow pattern of the hepatic vein
8. Evaluate feasibility of TV intervention

Tricuspid Valve Assessment: Due to the complexity of TV apparatus, multiple views should be used for imaging the TV leaflets, annulus and subvalvular apparatus. Ideally, both two-dimensional (2D) and three-dimensional (3D) imaging should be performed from multiple imaging windows to assess the anatomy. Off-axis imaging may be needed in patients where there is a massive RV or RA dilation. Recent studies have shed light on the variability in the number of TV leaflets, and efforts are underway to standardize the nomenclature of TV.[10] Evaluation of leaflet integrity and structure is critical while considering patients for TTVI. Three-dimensional imaging from transthoracic windows is often equivalent or better than TEE images due to the proximity of the probe to the valve. Narrow sector volumes focused on the valve from multiple views should be acquired.[48] Multibeat acquisition improves the frame rate and allows for direct planimetry of the regurgitant orifice area also known as vena contracta area. The approach to comprehensive assessment of the TV is addressed in the American Society of Echocardiography guidelines.[49,50]

Right Ventricular Assessment: Presence of concomitant right ventricular dysfunction with TR is considered high risk for any kind of TV intervention.[51,52] The vicious cycle of TR and right heart dysfunction is driven by the valvular pathologic condition. Progressive right heart failure often manifests as systemic venous congestion (edema, ascites), organ dysfunction (liver, kidney, bowel), and coagulopathy (hepatic and splenic dysfunction). Thorough assessment of RV function is critical at the time of TR assessment to help improve patient selection and determine optimal timing of intervention.

The conventional independent echocardiographic parameters used for the assessment of RV are tricuspid annular plane systolic excursion (TAPSE), fractional area change (FAC), RV myocardial performance index, lateral annulus peak systolic velocity (RV S′), and RV dP/dt. The comprehensive assessment of RV using these parameters is described in the ASE guidelines.[49] Newer echocardiographic methods of assessing RV function include RV strain, either free wall or global (including the septum)[53,54] and 3D RV ejection fraction[55,56] have been increasingly used clinically and have been associated with outcomes in patients with severe TR.[57–59]

In a compensated state, the RV adapts by increase in contractility with increasing afterload, whereas in decompensated state, RV function fails to increase. The assessment of RV contractile performance against the afterload by determining RV–PA coupling ratios provides important information regarding compensatory state of the RV and is a valuable prognostic marker in patients with HF with reduced ore preserved ejection fraction, PH as well as any valvular dysfunction.[60–64] The RV–PA coupling ratio is determined noninvasively by the ratio of TAPSE and echocardiographically derived PASP. TAPSE/PASP is associated with outcomes in patients with untreated secondary TR[65] as well as patients undergoing TTVI.[66] Recent analysis of the data from the TriValve registry also showed that patients whose RV–PA coupling ratio declined following TTVI had a better outcome compared with patients whose ratio did not change, suggesting that RV reserve may also be an important prognostic marker when considering TV intervention.[66]

Pulmonary Vascular Assessment: PH often coexists with significant TR and is associated with adverse outcomes following TV intervention.[18] Evaluation of baseline PASP is used to determine the preoperative risk. Echocardiographically determined PASP does not always correlate with invasive measurement, and therefore, combining invasive and echocardiographic PH assessment is necessary for preprocedural risk stratification. Recent study has shown that subjects with discordant invasive and echocardiographic PH have worst outcomes following

TTVI.[67,68] Echocardiographic parameters for RV assessment are summarized in Fig. 5.

Transesophageal echocardiogram (TEE): TEE examination done at various levels and multiplane angles allows for complete visualization and assessment of the TV apparatus and the RV. Additionally, careful assessment and quantification of left-sided pathologic condition, which may be contributing to this disease process, is also feasible. Visualization of the TV can be sometimes challenging by TEE in patients with horizontal heart, left-sided prosthesis, lipomatous interatrial septum, or atrial septal devices due to acoustic shadowing of the TV leaflets because the ultrasound beam crosses these structures. Although imaging from the midesophageal level, the esophagus is further away from the TV. Imaging from the distal esophagus

and the stomach allows for cleaner views of the TV because it is closer to the esophagus and hence the imaging probe. The guidelines for performing TEE by American Society of Echocardiography outline the key views for imaging the TV.[69,70] Ability to visualize the TV leaflets, subvalvular apparatus, and surrounding landmarks is crucial for TTVI. Three-dimensional imaging allows for careful delineation of the TV leaflets, aides in understanding the pathologic condition and allows for planning the interventional procedures.

The key views for TV and right heart evaluation by TTE and TEE are summarized in Figs. 6 and 7 respectively.

Intracardiac Imaging (ICE): ICE catheter is a narrow 3.0-mm tip (9 French) catheter that is introduced via the femoral vein and navigated

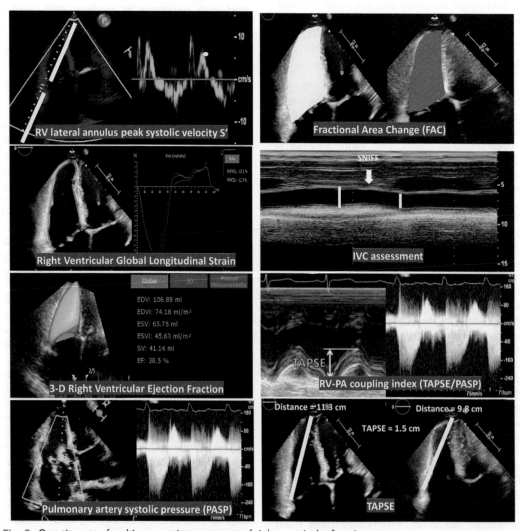

Fig. 5. Constituents of multiparametric assessment of right ventricular function.

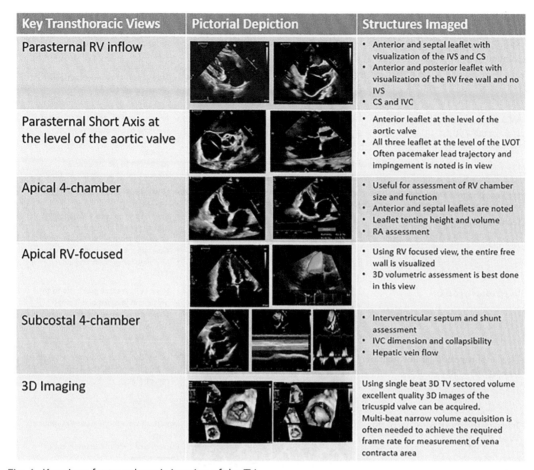

Key Transthoracic Views	Pictorial Depiction	Structures Imaged
Parasternal RV inflow		• Anterior and septal leaflet with visualization of the IVS and CS • Anterior and posterior leaflet with visualization of the RV free wall and no IVS • CS and IVC
Parasternal Short Axis at the level of the aortic valve		• Anterior leaflet at the level of the aortic valve • All three leaflet at the level of the LVOT • Often pacemaker lead trajectory and impingement is noted is in view
Apical 4-chamber		• Useful for assessment of RV chamber size and function • Anterior and septal leaflets are noted • Leaflet tenting height and volume • RA assessment
Apical RV-focused		• Using RV focused view, the entire free wall is visualized • 3D volumetric assessment is best done in this view
Subcostal 4-chamber		• Interventricular septum and shunt assessment • IVC dimension and collapsibility • Hepatic vein flow
3D Imaging		Using single beat 3D TV sectored volume excellent quality 3D images of the tricuspid valve can be acquired. Multi-beat narrow volume acquisition is often needed to achieve the required frame rate for measurement of vena contracta area

Fig. 6. Key views for transthoracic imaging of the TV.

to the heart for acquisition of high-quality 2D and 3D images in real-time. ICE during intraprocedural imaging is often used to supplement TEE imaging during transcatheter procedures. Acoustic shadowing from the delivery system or the prosthesis itself may lead to drop out with TEE imaging. ICE provides incremental value in such circumstances. The currently available 4D ICE catheters can obtain 2D and 3D volumetric images and cine-videos in real-time (4D) (Fig. 8). ICE has been proven to be a safe and efficacious modality for transcatheter electrophysiological as well as structural heart interventions.[71] Although currently used to complement the TEE imaging, in the future ICE may be used as a standalone device for imaging during TTVI.[72-75]

Multidetector Computed Tomography (MDCT): Specific acquisition protocols are needed for optimized imaging of the right heart and TV by MDCT. Type of scanner, left ventricular function, heart rate, presence of arrhythmia, renal function, and body habitus are key elements that should be accounted for while designing patient-specific protocol for the assessment of TR. Triphasic contrast bolus with contrast, mixture of saline/contrast and saline should be used.[76] Multiphasic cardiac-gated acquisition with imaging throughout the cardiac cycle must be attained to allow for postacquisition reconstruction from different phases. Cine imaging allows for the dynamic assessment of RV. Higher temporal resolution is achieved with dual source scanners or using multibeat acquisition with a single source scanner. RV volumes and function can be analyzed by semiautomated segmentation of the RV throughout the cardiac cycle. All 3 modalities have been shown to have excellent correlation in the assessment of RV function and volume.[77,78]

MDCT can provide characterization and precise measurements of the TA that help in sizing for TTVR. High temporal and spatial resolution also allow for the assessment of number of leaflets, delineation of TR cause (primary vs secondary), degree of prolapse/flail, extent of leaflet

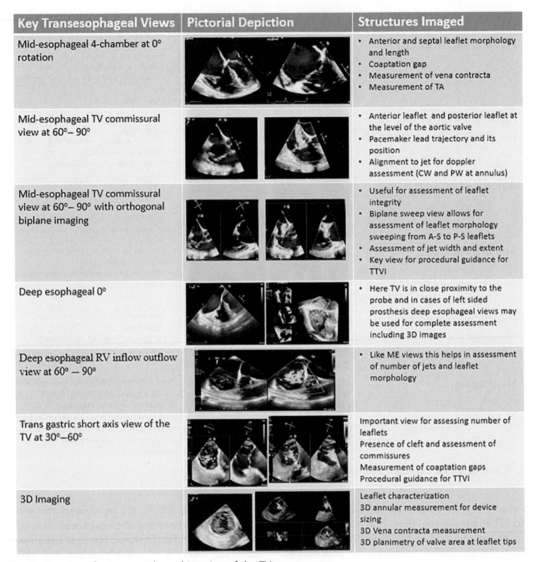

Key Transesophageal Views	Pictorial Depiction	Structures Imaged
Mid-esophageal 4-chamber at 0° rotation		• Anterior and septal leaflet morphology and length • Coaptation gap • Measurement of vena contracta • Measurement of TA
Mid-esophageal TV commissural view at 60°– 90°		• Anterior leaflet and posterior leaflet at the level of the aortic valve • Pacemaker lead trajectory and its position • Alignment to jet for doppler assessment (CW and PW at annulus)
Mid-esophageal TV commissural view at 60°– 90° with orthogonal biplane imaging		• Useful for assessment of leaflet integrity • Biplane sweep view allows for assessment of leaflet morphology sweeping from A-S to P-S leaflets • Assessment of jet width and extent • Key view for procedural guidance for TTVI
Deep esophageal 0°		• Here TV is in close proximity to the probe and in cases of left sided prosthesis deep esophageal views may be used for complete assessment including 3D images
Deep esophageal RV inflow outflow view at 60° – 90°		• Like ME views this helps in assessment of number of jets and leaflet morphology
Trans gastric short axis view of the TV at 30°–60°		Important view for assessing number of leaflets Presence of cleft and assessment of commissures Measurement of coaptation gaps Procedural guidance for TTVI
3D Imaging		Leaflet characterization 3D annular measurement for device sizing 3D Vena contracta measurement 3D planimetry of valve area at leaflet tips

Fig. 7. Key views for transesophageal imaging of the TV.

tenting, coaptation gap, as well as assessment of RA and RV chamber size (Fig. 9). Characterization of subvalvular apparatus and RV length and trabeculations are crucial to planning valvular intervention because certain devices need anchoring or clearance in the RV before deployment of the prosthesis. Retrograde opacification of IVC and hepatic veins with iodinated contrast is a specific marker of right heart disease and is often noted in patients with severe TR.[79] Unique to this modality is the benefit of planning of procedure by visualization of abdominal vasculature and access; accurate location and course of the right coronary artery in relation to the TA and assessment of the angulation between the IVC and TV.[80] Motion

and misintegration artifact are often seen in patients with atrial fibrillation. Newer generation multidetector scanners allow for shorter scan times and are less prone to artifact. Patient-specific protocol planning is key for acquiring the best possible dataset for comprehensive assessment of right heart pathologic condition.

Cardiac Magnetic Resonance (CMR): Accurate and reproducible assessment of RV function, wall motion abnormality, RV volume, and chamber quantification can be accomplished by CMR.[81,82] CMR plays a unique role in identifying right ventricular remodeling and fibrosis without the use of ionizing radiation. This imaging modality is the gold standard for tissue characterization. RV tissue characterization is

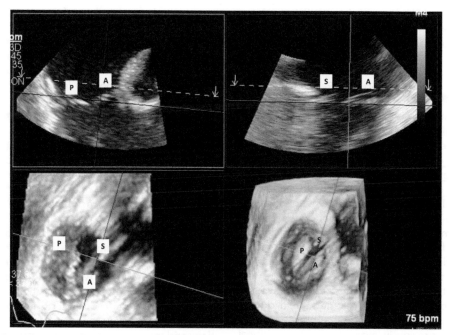

Fig. 8. Three-dimensional volumetric image of TV in real time using ICE catheter for procedural guidance.

possible using native T1 imaging and delayed gadolinium enhancement. Myocarditis, myocardial infarction, infiltrative disease, trauma, as well as PH can be differentiated using this modality. Regurgitant volume and regurgitant fraction for quantitative assessment of TR can be done using right-sided chamber volume along with phase contrast pulmonic flow. Short-axis cine images are typically used for volumetric measurements by tracing endocardial borders using semiautomated tracing techniques (see Fig. 9). Similar to MDCT, imaging protocols should account for the dilation of the RV and right atrium and include 4-chamber, RV inflow–

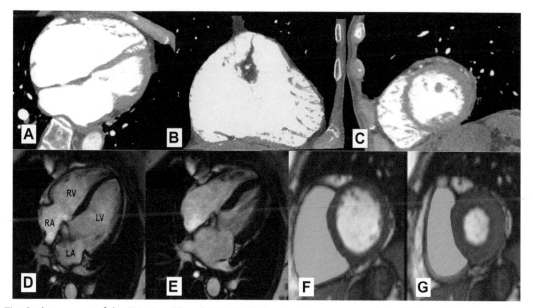

Fig. 9. Assessment of the RV using CT and MRI. (A–C) Anatomical assessment of the RV in multiple planes. (D, E) RV FAC assessment with MRI. (F, G) Endocardial tracing of short-axis cine images for the volumetric assessment of RV function.

outflow, and RV short axis images in its entirety. Leaflet length, tenting, prolapse, and thickening can all be assessed using sequential thin slice imaging.

CMR may be limited by arrhythmias, which often lead to motion artifact. Real-time cine imaging without breath-hold instructions are used in the patients with arrhythmia; however, the image resolution in such cases is suboptimal. Shortened free breathing real-time acquisition may be used to offset this problem. Presence of prosthetic devices and pacemaker leads may induce artifacts due to local magnetic field inhomogeneities. The interference of the magnetic field with the ferromagnetic material of the cardiac device may inadvertently lead to dislocation or loss of function. Historically, the presence of intracardiac device was considered as a contraindication to CMR. However, efforts are underway to transition to CMR-safe devices that have less interaction between the magnetic field due to reduced amount of ferromagnetic material from the previously available CMR-conditional and CMR-unsafe devices. CMR conditional pacemakers have been commercially available since 2011 and majority of the patient population we deal with have these devices. The devices should be reprogrammed to prevent inappropriate activation or shock, and typically, CMR sequences with a specific absorption rate of 2.0 W/kg or lesser should be used.[83] Several techniques have been developed to avoid image artifacts, these include the use of imaging planes perpendicular to the plane of the cardiac device, inversion and excitation pulses bandwidth widening, echo time shortening, and the implementation of a frequency scout before steady-state free precession sequences or the use of spoiled gradient echo cine imaging.[84–86]

NOVEL TREATMENT STRATEGIES

Current guideline-directed medical treatment includes a IIa recommendation for diuretics, aimed at reducing the preload; however, the level of evidence (Category C) remains limited.[3] Guidelines also give a IIa recommendation for the treatment of left heart disease and PH, which is aimed at reducing the afterload. Although the evidence is also limited for this recommendation, recent studies suggest that the reduction of mitral regurgitation with TEER[87] and cardiac resynchronization therapy for left heart failure[88] may be effective in reducing TR and improving outcomes. Recurrent heart failure hospitalizations and mortality remains high despite medical therapy. Based on degree of regurgitation and presence of symptoms various stages of TR have been defined by the recent The American College of Cardiology and American Heart Association (ACC/AHA) guidelines for the management of valvular heart disease.

Stage B represents progressive TR, quantified as nonsevere without any hemodynamic consequences. Stage C is asymptomatic severe TR with hemodynamic consequences like dilated

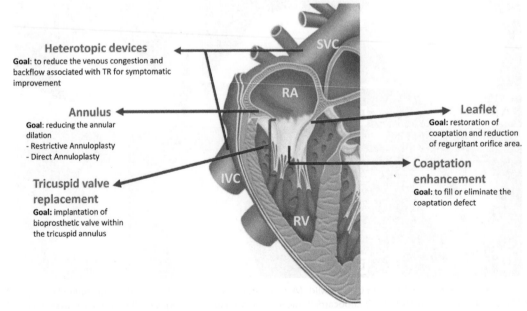

Fig. 10. Targets of current transcatheter TV therapy.

Table 2
Current devices under investigation for transcatheter tricuspid valve intervention

Device Target	Current Devices	Useful Imaging Modalities	Advantages	Limitations
Annulus Goal: reducing the annular dilation	Restrictive Annuloplasty • TRIAPTA (transatrial intrapericardial tricuspid annuloplasty) Direct Annuloplasty • Cardioband (Edwards Lifesciences) • MIA-T (Micro Interventional Devices, Inc) • DaVingi (Cardiac Implants LLC)	Baseline: CT • Annular sizing - location of RCA; TEE for baseline annular sizing and quantification of regurgitation and chamber dimensions; Intraprocedural: TEE and ICE for intraprocedural guidance; Postprocedure: TTE and CT for postprocedural follow-up	Useful for regurgitation due to annular dilatation; Useful in atrial functional TR	• In investigational stages • Challenges with anchor deployment along the ill-defined tricuspid annulus • Proximity of the RCA to the annulus may prove to be a limitation
Leaflet Goal: restoration of coaptation and reduction of regurgitant orifice area	• TriClip (Abbott Vascular, Santa Clara, Ca) • PASCAL (Edwards Lifesciences)	Baseline: TTE and TEE: For quantification of regurgitation and assessment of leaflet morphology and coaptation gaps. CT may also be helpful in measurement of coaptation gap; Intraprocedural: TEE and ICE for intraprocedural guidance; Postprocedure: TTE with 3D assessment of prosthesis	• Most experience among tricuspid devices • No need for full anticoagulation postimplantation unlike valve replacement	• Procedural learning curve • Incomplete reduction of TR • Not ideal for regurgitation with large central coaptation gaps • Not ideal for multiple regurgitant jets
Coaptation enhancement Goal: to fill or eliminate the coaptation defect	• DUO • TriFlo	TEE/CT or MRI	• Ideal for patients with large central coaptation defects	

(continued on next page)

Table 2
(continued)

Device Target	Current Devices	Useful Imaging Modalities	Advantages	Limitations
TV replacement Goal: implantation of bioprosthetic valve within the tricuspid annulus	• EVOQUE system (Edwards Lifesciences) • LuX-Valve (Ningbo Jenscare Biotechnology, China) • Intrepid (Medtronic) • Tricares • Trisol • V-Dyne • Cardiovalve	Baseline: TEE/TTE: For quantification of regurgitation and assessment of leaflet morphology and annular measurement. RV assessment CT is mainstay for annular measurement and sizing Intraprocedural: TEE and ICE for intraprocedural guidance Postprocedure: TTE with 3D assessment of prosthesis. CT for prosthetic valve dysfunction and RV assessment	• Complete elimination of TR • Ideal for patients with large coaptation gaps	• Limited data on long-term durability • Management of RV dysfunction postprocedure may be challenging • It is unclear who the ideal candidates for this therapy would be
Heterotopic devices Goal: to reduce the venous congestion and backflow associated with TR for symptomatic improvement	• TricValve (P&F products Features Vertriebs, Vienna, Austria) • Tricento (NVT GmBH Hechingen, Germany) • Caval SAPIEN 3 (Edwards Lifesciences)	Baseline: CT: Measurement of the IVC and SVC dimensions Intraprocedural: TEE and TTE: To assess landing zones of the valves Fluoroscopy is used as adjunctive imaging Postprocedure: TTE	• May be the only option currently available for patients with severe annular dilatation who do not make the inclusion criteria for TTVR and have large coaptation gaps, which make them poor candidate for TEER therapy	• Little or no effect on immediate right heart hemodynamics • Cannot be used for patients with severe caval enlargement

TR Patient's Journey

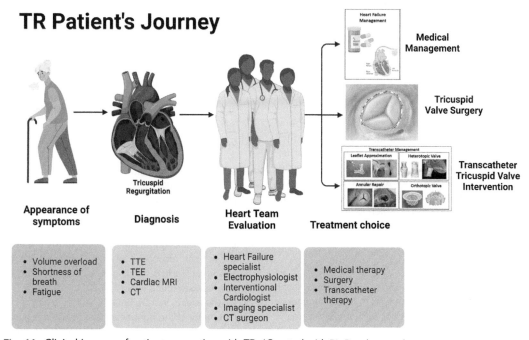

Fig. 11. Clinical journey of patient presenting with TR. (*Created with* BioRender.com.)

RA/RV with elevated right sided pressures, but no patient reported symptoms. Stage D is symptomatic severe TR, with hemodynamic consequences and patient reported symptoms.

Both ACC/AHA guidelines and ESC/EACTS guidelines[89] recommend surgical intervention for severe primary or secondary TR at the time of left-sided intervention for patients with Stage C or D (Class I) and to prevent the progression of secondary disease in Stage B patients who exhibit TA dilatation of more than 4 cm and/or RV dysfunction (Class IIa). TV surgery for isolated primary TR received a IIa indication for Stage D and IIb for Stage C. Patients with secondary TR attributable to annular dilatation (without PH or left-sided disease) who are poorly responsive to medical therapy, TV surgery is a Class IIa indication. Surgery however was favored in the ESC and EACTS recommendations that gave it a Class 1 for isolated severe primary TR without severe RV dysfunction.[89]

The key to ensure positive outcomes is patient selection. Severely reduced RV function, congestive hepatopathy, and multiorgan dysfunction often are markers for poor outcomes. The advent of transcatheter therapy is a promising new approach to manage this challenging patient population. The targets of current TV therapy are demonstrated in Fig. 10. The treatment of severe TR with transcatheter edge-to-edge repair (TEER) therapy is recognized as 2b recommendation by 2021 ESC/

ECATS due to Conformité Européene approved tricuspid TEER device in inoperable patients at a comprehensive heart center with expertise. The current devices under investigation are listed in Table 2.

There are several challenges with designing trials for the treatment of TV disease using minimally invasive transcatheter approach. Standardization of patient selection criteria based on preprocedural imaging and clinical assessment is needed to warrant positive outcomes. Identifying goals of therapy upfront is critical and would play a crucial role in device selection. Ideal timing of intervention to ensure best possible outcomes is yet to be defined. Early recognition, referral, and timely intervention may prevent the progression to refractory right heart failure, RV chamber dilation, and end-organ dysfunction (Fig. 11).

CLINICS CARE POINTS

- Before consideration of invasive intervention, optimization of hemodynamic state has shown to improve outcomes.

- In the presence of CIED, look for device impingement on the TV apparatus.

- Involve heart failure team right from the time of initial assessment and diagnosis.

DISCLOSURE

Dr V Agarwal reports speaker fees from Abbott Structural; she has a consulting agreement with ReNiva Inc. and Moray medical. Dr R. Hahn reports speaker fees from Abbott Structural, Baylis Medical, Edwards Lifesciences, and Philips Healthcare; she has institutional consulting contracts for which she receives no direct compensation with Abbott Structural, Boston Scientific, Edwards Lifesciences, Medtronic and Novartis; she is Chief Scientific Officer for the Echocardiography Core Laboratory at the Cardiovascular Research Foundation for multiple industry-sponsored TV trials, for which she receives no direct industry compensation.

REFERENCES

1. Dreyfus GD, Martin RP, Chan KM, et al. Functional tricuspid regurgitation: a need to revise our understanding. J Am Coll Cardiol 2015;65:2331–6.

2. Topilsky Y, Maltais S, Medina Inojosa J, et al. Burden of Tricuspid Regurgitation in Patients Diagnosed in the Community Setting. JACC Cardiovasc Imaging 2019;12:433–42.

3. Otto CM, Nishimura RA, Bonow RO, et al. 2020 ACC/AHA Guideline for the Management of Patients With Valvular Heart Disease: A Report of the American College of Cardiology/American Heart Association Joint, Committee on Clinical Practice Guidelines. J Am Coll Cardiol 2021;77: e25–197.

4. Dahou A, Levin D, Reisman M, et al. Anatomy and Physiology of the Tricuspid Valve. JACC Cardiovasc Imaging 2019;12:458–68.

5. Addetia K, Muraru D, Veronesi F, et al. 3-Dimensional Echocardiographic Analysis of the Tricuspid Annulus Provides New Insights Into Tricuspid Valve Geometry and Dynamics. J Am Coll Cardiol 2017; 12(3):401–12.

6. Messer S, Moseley E, Marinescu M, et al. Histologic analysis of the right atrioventricular junction in the adult human heart. J Heart Valve Dis 2012;21: 368–73.

7. El-Busaid H, Hassan S, Odula P, et al. Sex variations in the structure of human atrioventricular annuli. Folia Morphol (Warsz) 2012;71:23–7.

8. Singh JP, Evans JC, Levy D, et al. Prevalence and clinical determinants of mitral, tricuspid, and aortic regurgitation (the Framingham Heart Study). Am J Cardiol 1999;83:897–902.

9. Naser JA, Pislaru C, Roslan A, et al. Unfavorable Tricuspid Annulus Dynamics: A Novel Concept to Explain Development of Tricuspid Regurgitation in Atrial Fibrillation. J Am Soc Echocardiogr 2022; 35:664–6.

10. Hahn RT, Weckbach LT, Noack T, et al. Proposal for a Standard Echocardiographic Tricuspid Valve Nomenclature. JACC Cardiovasc Imaging 2021; 14(7):1299–305.

11. Haddad F, Hunt SA, Rosenthal DN, et al. Right ventricular function in cardiovascular disease, part I: Anatomy, physiology, aging, and functional assessment of the right ventricle. Circulation 2008;117: 1436–48.

12. Sanz J, Sánchez-Quintana D, Bossone E, et al. Anatomy, Function, and Dysfunction of the Right Ventricle: JACC State-of-the-Art Review. J Am Coll Cardiol 2019;73:1463–82.

13. MacNee W. Pathophysiology of cor pulmonale in chronic obstructive pulmonary disease. Part One. Am J Respir Crit Care Med 1994;150:833–52.

14. Bartelds B, Borgdorff MA, Smit-van Oosten A, et al. Differential responses of the right ventricle to abnormal loading conditions in mice: pressure vs. volume load. Eur J Heart Fail 2011;13:1275–82.

15. De Meester P, Van De Bruaene A, Herijgers P, et al. Geometry of the right heart and tricuspid regurgitation to exclude elevated pulmonary artery pressure: new insights. Int J Cardiol 2013;168:3866–71.

16. Vonk-Noordegraaf A, Haddad F, Chin KM, et al. Right heart adaptation to pulmonary arterial hypertension: physiology and pathobiology. J Am Coll Cardiol 2013;62:D22–33.

17. Spinner EM, Lerakis S, Higginson J, et al. Correlates of tricuspid regurgitation as determined by 3D echocardiography: pulmonary arterial pressure, ventricle geometry, annular dilatation, and papillary muscle displacement. Circ Cardiovasc Imaging 2012;5:43–50.

18. Kim YJ, Kwon DA, Kim HK, et al. Determinants of surgical outcome in patients with isolated tricuspid regurgitation. Circulation 2009;120:1672–8.

19. Muraru D, Addetia K, Guta AC, et al. Right atrial volume is a major determinant of tricuspid annulus area in functional tricuspid regurgitation: a three-dimensional echocardiographic study. Eur Heart J Cardiovasc Imaging 2021;22:660–9.

20. Utsunomiya H, Itabashi Y, Mihara H, et al. Functional Tricuspid Regurgitation Caused by Chronic Atrial Fibrillation: A Real-Time 3-Dimensional Transesophageal Echocardiography Study. Circ Cardiovasc Imaging 2017;10.

21. Mutlak D, Khalil J, Lessick J, et al. Risk Factors for the Development of Functional Tricuspid Regurgitation and Their Population-Attributable Fractions. JACC Cardiovasc Imaging 2020;13:1643–51.

22. Praz F, Muraru D, Kreidel F, et al. Transcatheter treatment for tricuspid valve disease. EuroIntervention 2021;17:791–808.

23. Lancellotti P, Pibarot P, Chambers J, et al. Multimodality imaging assessment of native valvular regurgitation: an EACVI and ESC council of valvular

heart disease position paper. Eur Heart J Cardiovasc Imaging 2022;23(5):e171–232.

24. Addetia K, Harb SC, Hahn RT, et al. Cardiac Implantable Electronic Device Lead-Induced Tricuspid Regurgitation. JACC Cardiovasc Imaging 2019;12:622–36.

25. Zhang XX, Wei M, Xiang R, et al. Incidence, Risk Factors, and Prognosis of Tricuspid Regurgitation After Cardiac Implantable Electronic Device Implantation: A Systematic Review and Meta-analysis. J Cardiothorac Vasc Anesth 2022;36:1741–55.

26. Hoke U, Auger D, Thijssen J, et al. Significant lead-induced tricuspid regurgitation is associated with poor prognosis at long-term follow-up. Heart 2014;100:960–8.

27. Delling FN, Hassan ZK, Piatkowski G, et al. Tricuspid Regurgitation and Mortality in Patients With Transvenous Permanent Pacemaker Leads. Am J Cardiol 2016;117:988–92.

28. Prihadi EA, van der Bijl P, Gursoy E, et al. Development of significant tricuspid regurgitation over time and prognostic implications: new insights into natural history. Eur Heart J 2018;39:3574–81.

29. Arsalan M, Walther T, Smith RL 2nd, et al. Tricuspid regurgitation diagnosis and treatment. Eur Heart J 2017;38:634–8.

30. Badano LP, Muraru D, Enriquez-Sarano M. Assessment of functional tricuspid regurgitation. Eur Heart J 2013;34:1875–85.

31. Muraru D, Guta AC, Ochoa-Jimenez RC, et al. Functional Regurgitation of Atrioventricular Valves and Atrial Fibrillation: An Elusive Pathophysiological Link Deserving Further Attention. J Am Soc Echocardiogr 2020;33:42–53.

32. Florescu DR, Muraru D, Volpato V, et al. Atrial Functional Tricuspid Regurgitation as a Distinct Pathophysiological and Clinical Entity: No Idiopathic Tricuspid Regurgitation Anymore. J Clin Med 2022;11:382.

33. Delgado V, Bax JJ. Atrial Functional Mitral Regurgitation: From Mitral Annulus Dilatation to Insufficient Leaflet Remodeling. Circ Cardiovasc Imaging 2017; 10:e006239.

34. Zoghbi WA, Levine RA, Flachskampf F, et al. Atrial Functional Mitral Regurgitation: A JACC: Cardiovascular Imaging Expert Panel Viewpoint. JACC Cardiovasc Imaging 2022;15:1870–82.

35. Schlotter F, Dietz MF, Stolz L, et al. Atrial Functional Tricuspid Regurgitation: Novel Definition and Impact on Prognosis. Circ Cardiovasc Interv 2022;15:e011958.

36. Vahanian A, Beyersdorf F, Praz F, et al. 2021 ESC/EACTS Guidelines for the management of valvular heart disease: Developed by the Task Force for the management of valvular heart disease of the European Society of Cardiology (ESC) and the European Association for Cardio-Thoracic Surgery (EACTS). Eur Heart J 2021;75(6):524.

37. Muraru D, Caravita S, Guta AC, et al. Functional Tricuspid Regurgitation and Atrial Fibrillation: Which Comes First, the Chicken or the Egg? CASE (Philadelphia, Pa) 2020;4:458–63.

38. Badano LP, Caravita S, Rella V, et al. The Added Value of 3-Dimensional Echocardiography to Understand the Pathophysiology of Functional Tricuspid Regurgitation. JACC Cardiovasc Imaging 2021;14:683–9.

39. Topilsky Y, Inojosa JM, Benfari G, et al. Clinical presentation and outcome of tricuspid regurgitation in patients with systolic dysfunction. Eur Heart J 2018; 39:3584–92.

40. Topilsky Y, Nkomo VT, Vatury O, et al. Clinical outcome of isolated tricuspid regurgitation. JACC Cardiovasc Imaging 2014;7:1185–94.

41. Poelzl G, Auer J. Cardiohepatic syndrome. Curr Heart Fail Rep 2015;12:68–78.

42. Stolz L, Orban M, Besler C, et al. Cardiohepatic Syndrome Is Associated With Poor Prognosis in Patients Undergoing Tricuspid Transcatheter Edge-to-Edge Valve Repair. JACC Cardiovasc Interv 2022;15:179–89.

43. House AA, Anand I, Bellomo R, et al. Definition and classification of Cardio-Renal Syndromes: workgroup statements from the 7th ADQI Consensus Conference. Nephrol Dial Transplant 2010;25: 1416–20.

44. Hewing B, Mattig I, Knebel F, et al. Renal and hepatic function of patients with severe tricuspid regurgitation undergoing inferior caval valve implantation. Sci Rep 2021;11:21800.

45. Lauten A, Figulla HR, Unbehaun A, et al. Interventional Treatment of Severe Tricuspid Regurgitation: Early Clinical Experience in a Multicenter, Observational, First-in-Man Study. Circ Cardiovasc Interv 2018;11:e006061.

46. Karam N, Braun D, Mehr M, et al. Impact of Transcatheter Tricuspid Valve Repair for Severe Tricuspid Regurgitation on Kidney and Liver Function. JACC Cardiovasc Interv 2019;12:1413–20.

47. Lancellotti P, Tribouilloy C, Hagendorff A, et al. Recommendations for the echocardiographic assessment of native valvular regurgitation: an executive summary from the European Association of Cardiovascular Imaging. Eur Heart J Cardiovasc Imaging 2013;14:611–44.

48. Muraru D, Hahn RT, Soliman OI, et al. 3-Dimensional Echocardiography in Imaging the Tricuspid Valve. JACC Cardiovasc Imaging 2019;12:500–15.

49. Rudski LG, Lai WW, Afilalo J, et al. Guidelines for the echocardiographic assessment of the right heart in adults: a report from the American Society of Echocardiography endorsed by the European Association of Echocardiography, a registered branch of the European Society of Cardiology, and the Canadian Society of Echocardiography.

J Am Soc Echocardiogr 2010;23:685–713 [quiz: 786–8].

50. Lang RM, Badano LP, Tsang W, et al. EAE/ASE recommendations for image acquisition and display using three-dimensional echocardiography. J Am Soc Echocardiogr 2012;25:3–46.

51. Elgharably H, Ibrahim A, Rosinski B, et al. Right heart failure and patient selection for isolated tricuspid valve surgery. J Thorac Cardiovasc Surg 2021. https://doi.org/10.1016/j.jtcvs.2021.10.059.

52. Taramasso M, Alessandrini H, Latib A, et al. Outcomes After Current Transcatheter Tricuspid Valve Intervention: Mid-Term Results From the International TriValve Registry. JACC Cardiovasc Interv 2019;12:155–65.

53. Muraru D, Haugaa K, Donal E, et al. Right ventricular longitudinal strain in the clinical routine: a state-of-the-art review. Eur Heart J Cardiovasc Imaging 2022;23:898–912.

54. Addetia K, Miyoshi T, Citro R, et al. Two-Dimensional Echocardiographic Right Ventricular Size and Systolic Function Measurements Stratified by Sex, Age, and Ethnicity: Results of the World Alliance of Societies of Echocardiography Study. J Am Soc Echocardiogr 2021;34:1148–57.e1.

55. Namisaki H, Nabeshima Y, Kitano T, et al. Prognostic Value of the Right Ventricular Ejection Fraction, Assessed by Fully Automated Three-Dimensional Echocardiography: A Direct Comparison of Analyses Using Right Ventricular-Focused Views versus Apical Four-Chamber Views. J Am Soc Echocardiogr 2021;34:117–26.

56. Muraru D, Badano LP, Nagata Y, et al. Development and prognostic validation of partition values to grade right ventricular dysfunction severity using 3D echocardiography. Eur Heart J Cardiovasc Imaging 2020;21:10–21.

57. Prihadi EA, van der Bijl P, Dietz M, et al. Prognostic Implications of Right Ventricular Free Wall Longitudinal Strain in Patients With Significant Functional Tricuspid Regurgitation. Circ Cardiovasc Imaging 2019;12:e008666.

58. Kresoja KP, Rommel KP, Lücke C, et al. Right Ventricular Contraction Patterns in Patients Undergoing Transcatheter Tricuspid Valve Repair for Severe Tricuspid Regurgitation. JACC Cardiovasc Interv 2021;1551–61.

59. Orban M, Wolff S, Braun D, et al. Right Ventricular Function in Transcatheter Edge-to-Edge Tricuspid Valve Repair. J Am Coll Cardiol 2021;14:2477–9.

60. Bosch L, Lam CSP, Gong L, et al. Right ventricular dysfunction in left-sided heart failure with preserved versus reduced ejection fraction. Eur J Heart Fail 2017;19:1664–71.

61. Melenovsky V, Hwang SJ, Lin G, et al. Right heart dysfunction in heart failure with preserved ejection fraction. Eur Heart J 2014;35:3452–62.

62. Hsu S, Simpson CE, Houston BA, et al. Multi-Beat Right Ventricular-Arterial Coupling Predicts Clinical Worsening in Pulmonary Arterial Hypertension. J Am Heart Assoc 2020;9:e016031.

63. Vanderpool RR, Pinsky MR, Naeije R, et al. RV-pulmonary arterial coupling predicts outcome in patients referred for pulmonary hypertension. Heart 2015;101:37–43.

64. Eleid MF, Padang R, Pislaru SV, et al. Effect of Transcatheter Aortic Valve Replacement on Right Ventricular-Pulmonary Artery Coupling. JACC Cardiovasc Interv 2019;12:2145–54.

65. Fortuni F, Butcher SC, Dietz MF, et al. Right Ventricular-Pulmonary Arterial Coupling in Secondary Tricuspid Regurgitation. Am J Cardiol 2021;148:138–45.

66. Brener MI, Lurz P, Hausleiter J, et al. Right Ventricular-Pulmonary Arterial Coupling and Afterload Reserve in Patients Undergoing Transcatheter Tricuspid Valve Repair. J Am Coll Cardiol 2022;79:448–61.

67. Lurz P, Orban M, Besler C, et al. Clinical characteristics, diagnosis, and risk stratification of pulmonary hypertension in severe tricuspid regurgitation and implications for transcatheter tricuspid valve repair. Eur Heart J 2020;41:2785–95.

68. Hahn RT. Finding concordance in discord: the value of discordant invasive and echocardiographic pulmonary artery pressure measurements with severe tricuspid regurgitation. Eur Heart J 2020;41:2796–8.

69. Hahn RT, Abraham T, Adams MS, et al. Guidelines for performing a comprehensive transesophageal echocardiographic examination: recommendations from the American Society of Echocardiography and the Society of Cardiovascular Anesthesiologists. J Am Soc Echocardiogr 2013;26:921–64.

70. Hahn RT, Saric M, Faletra FF, et al. Recommended Standards for the Performance of Transesophageal Echocardiographic Screening for Structural Heart Intervention: From the American Society of Echocardiography. J Am Soc Echocardiogr 2022;35:1–76.

71. Hagemeyer D, Ali FM, Ong G, et al. The Role of Intracardiac Echocardiography in Percutaneous Tricuspid Intervention: A New ICE Age. Interv Cardiol Clin 2022;11:103–12.

72. Møller JE, De Backer O, Nuyens P, et al. Transesophageal and intracardiac echocardiography to guide transcatheter tricuspid valve repair with the TriClip™ system. Int J Cardiovasc Imaging 2022;38:609–11.

73. Curio J, Abulgasim K, Kasner M, et al. Intracardiac echocardiography to enable successful edge-to-edge transcatheter tricuspid valve repair in patients with insufficient TEE quality. Clin Hemorheol Microcirc 2020;76:199–210.

74. Wong I, Chui ASF, Wong CY, et al. Complimentary Role of ICE and TEE During Transcatheter Edge-to-Edge Tricuspid Valve Repair With TriClip G4. JACC Cardiovasc Interv 2022;15:562–3.

75. Davidson CJ, Abramson S, Smith RL, et al. Transcatheter Tricuspid Repair With the Use of 4-Dimensional Intracardiac Echocardiography. JACC Cardiovasc Imaging 2022;15:533–8.

76. Hinzpeter R, Eberhard M, Burghard P, et al. Computed tomography in patients with tricuspid regurgitation prior to transcatheter valve repair: dynamic analysis of the annulus with an individually tailored contrast media protocol. EuroIntervention 2017;12:e1828–36.

77. Henneman MM, Schuijf JD, Jukema JW, et al. Assessment of global and regional left ventricular function and volumes with 64-slice MSCT: a comparison with 2D echocardiography. J Nucl Cardiol 2006;13:480–7.

78. Greupner J, Zimmermann E, Grohmann A, et al. Head-to-head comparison of left ventricular function assessment with 64-row computed tomography, biplane left cineventriculography, and both 2- and 3-dimensional transthoracic echocardiography: comparison with magnetic resonance imaging as the reference standard. J Am Coll Cardiol 2012;59:1897–907.

79. Yeh BM, Kurzman P, Foster E, et al. Clinical relevance of retrograde inferior vena cava or hepatic vein opacification during contrast-enhanced CT. AJR Am J Roentgenol 2004;183:1227–32.

80. Prihadi EA, Delgado V, Hahn RT, et al. Imaging Needs in Novel Transcatheter Tricuspid Valve Interventions. JACC Cardiovasc Imaging 2018;11:736–54.

81. Koch JA, Poll LW, Godehardt E, et al. Right and left ventricular volume measurements in an animal heart model in vitro: first experiences with cardiac MRI at 1.0 T. Eur Radiol 2000;10:455–8.

82. Jauhiainen T, Jarvinen VM, Hekali PE, et al. MR gradient echo volumetric analysis of human cardiac casts: focus on the right ventricle. J Comput Assist Tomogr 1998;22:899–903.

83. Baker KB, Tkach JA, Nyenhuis JA, et al. Evaluation of specific absorption rate as a dosimeter of MRI-related implant heating. J Magn Reson Imaging 2004;20:315–20.

84. Olivieri LJ, Cross RR, O'Brien KE, et al. Optimized protocols for cardiac magnetic resonance imaging in patients with thoracic metallic implants. Pediatr Radiol 2015;45:1455–64.

85. Rashid S, Rapacchi S, Vaseghi M, et al. Improved late gadolinium enhancement MR imaging for patients with implanted cardiac devices. Radiology 2014;270:269–74.

86. Symons R, Zimmerman SL, Bluemke DA. CMR and CT of the Patient With Cardiac Devices: Safety, Efficacy, and Optimization Strategies. JACC Cardiovasc Imaging 2019;12:890–903.

87. Hahn RT, Asch F, Weissman NJ, et al. Impact of Tricuspid Regurgitation on Clinical Outcomes: The COAPT Trial. J Am Coll Cardiol 2020;76:1305–14.

88. Stassen J, Galloo X, Hirasawa K, et al. Tricuspid regurgitation after cardiac resynchronization therapy: evolution and prognostic significance. Europace 2022;24:1291–9.

89. Vahanian A, Beyersdorf F, Praz F, et al. 2021 ESC/EACTS Guidelines for the management of valvular heart disease. Eur Heart J 2022;43:561–632.

Multimodality Imaging in Aortic Stenosis
Beyond the Valve - Focusing on the Myocardium

Safwan Gaznabi, MD[a,b], Jeirym Miranda, MD[a,c],
Daniel Lorenzatti, MD[a], Pamela Piña, MD[a,d],
Senthil S. Balasubramanian, MD[b], Darshi Desai, MD[e],
Aditya Desai, MD[e], Edwin C. Ho, MD[a],
Andrea Scotti, MD[a], Carlos A. Gongora, MD[a],
Aldo L. Schenone, MD[a], Mario J. Garcia, MD[a],
Azeem Latib, MD[a], Purvi Parwani, MBBS, MPH[f],
Leandro Slipczuk, MD, PhD[a,*]

KEYWORDS

- Aortic stenosis • Low flow low gradient • Discordant • Asymptomatic
- Global longitudinal strain • Fibrosis • Myocardium

KEY POINTS

- Aortic stenosis is a complex, multifaceted disease leading to myocardial remodeling and ultimately to heart failure or sudden death.
- Traditional focus is shifting from the valve alone to integrate the myocardium through the evaluation of subclinical left ventricle remodeling and myocardial fibrosis to identify the best timing for aortic valve replacement (AVR).
- Echocardiography-driven cardiac damage and myocardial deformation parameters (global longitudinal strain and left atrium strain) are independently associated with outcomes pre- and post-AVR.
- Cardiovascular magnetic resonance evaluation can predict outcomes based on the evaluation of reversible interstitial fibrosis (increased T1/ extracellular volume) and irreversible replacement fibrosis (late gadolinium enhancement).
- Cardiac computed tomography allows for the evaluation of myocardial deformation, interstitial fibrosis, and advanced valve characterization.

This article originally appeared in *Heart Failure Clinics*, Volume 19 Issue 4, October 2023.
[a] Division of Cardiology, Montefiore Medical Center/Albert Einstein College of Medicine, 111 East 210th street, Bronx, NY 10467, USA; [b] Division of Cardiology, University of Chicago at Northshore University Health System, 1000 Central Street, Evanston, IL 60201, USA; [c] Division of Cardiology, Mount Sinai Morningside. 419 West 114th Street, NY 10025, USA; [d] Division of Cardiology, CEDIMAT. Arturo Logroño, Plaza de la Salud, Dr. Juan Manuel Taveras Rodríguez, C. Pepillo Salcedo esq. Santo Domingo, Dominican Republic; [e] Department of Internal Medicine, University of California Riverside School of Medicine. 900 University Avenue, Riverside, CA 92521, USA; [f] Division of Cardiology, Department of Medicine, Loma Linda University Health, 11234 Anderson Street, Loma Linda, CA 92354, USA
* Corresponding author. Division of Cardiology, Montefiore Medical Center, 111 East 210th street, Bronx, NY 10467.
E-mail address: lslipczukb@montefiore.org

BEYOND A VALVE-FOCUSED ASSESSMENT AND MANAGEMENT OF AORTIC STENOSIS

Aortic stenosis (AS) is a progressive and potentially fatal disease that leads to an increased afterload of the left ventricle (LV), subsequent myocardial remodeling, and heart failure.[1] With an estimated 12.6 million cases globally reported in 2017, AS is the third most common cardiovascular disease in the United States and Europe, with an increasing prevalence of up to 7% in those greater than 65 years of age.[2] The most common etiology is the fibrocalcific thickening of the aortic valve leaflets leading to progressive restricted leaflet opening, with less common etiologies being congenital bicuspid, rheumatic fever, and radiation.[3] It is well-established that severe AS patients who develop symptoms or impaired left ventricular ejection fraction (LVEF) have poor outcomes without aortic valve replacement (AVR).[4] Even though a traditional focus has been on the aortic valve itself, the recent demonstration of subclinical LV remodeling and myocardial fibrosis, together with increased events in patients with traditionally nonsevere AS, has shifted the attention to the myocardium as a complementary marker of the disease process.[5,6] In this review, the authors summarize the available data on the use of multimodality imaging in evaluating the interplay between severe AS and myocardial characterization for risk stratification of patients with AS (Fig. 1).

The current 2020 American Heart Association/American College of Cardiology (AHA/ACC) guidelines emphasize a comprehensive assessment of AS and recommend AVR when symptoms or overt myocardial systolic dysfunction (LVEF <50%) ensue. From the initial valve-centered risk stratification, Genereux and colleagues developed an extravalvular staging classification based on cardiac damage. In patients from the PARTNER 2 trial, the stage of cardiac damage by echocardiography was independently associated with increased mortality after AVR (HR 1.46 per each increment in stage, $P<.0001$).[7] Utilization of multimodality imaging techniques such as echocardiography with global longitudinal strain (GLS), PET, cardiac computed tomography (CT) (Fig. 2), and cardiovascular magnetic resonance (CMR) imaging (Fig. 3) have provided a wealth of information as to myocardial remodeling secondary to AS. This approach is nevertheless not routinely implemented nor clearly defined in guideline-directed practice for AS, as opposed to regurgitant disease.[4,8]

CHALLENGES OF DISCORDANT ECHOCARDIOGRAPHIC FINDINGS

An accurate assessment of AS severity is crucial for optimal management and timing of AVR. Echocardiography, including Doppler evaluation, is the gold standard imaging modality for grading AS severity, allowing a comprehensive structural and hemodynamic evaluation of the aortic valve and the LV myocardial response, including hypertrophy, remodeling, and ejection fraction. Concordant severe AS is defined in its typical form of high-gradient (HG)-AS as an aortic valve area (AVA) less than 1.0 cm^2 or an indexed AVA (AVAi) less than 0.6 cm^2/m^2 and maximum velocity greater than 4 m/s or a mean gradient greater than 40 mm Hg.[9,10] However, up to 40% of patients present with "discordant grading" on Doppler echocardiography, and it is also referred to as "low-gradient AS," defined as an AVA consistent with severe (<1.0 cm^2 and <0.6 cm^2/m^2) but with a low gradient/velocity (<40 mm Hg, <4 m/s). In this situation, one must first rule out measurement or calculation errors. Other known sources of error are the poor alignment of the ultrasound beam, the neglect of elevated subvalvular velocities, and the occurrence of pressure recovery.[11]

This discordant pattern may raise uncertainties regarding the true severity of the valve disease and its therapeutic management.[10] The stroke volume index (SVi) is a marker of LV systolic function and an important prognostic factor before and after AVR. Furthermore, because the mean gradient is not only directly related to the stroke volume but also inversely related to the ejection time, a definition of a low-flow state as a mean flow rate less than 200 mL/s has been suggested and associated with a worse prognosis and with a higher likelihood of "pseudo-moderate" gradient and/or pseudo-severe AVA.[12] The discordant low-gradient severe AS entity includes (1) classical low flow (SVi < 35 mL/m^2), low gradient with reduced LVEF (LVEF < 50%); (2) paradoxical low-flow, low-gradient AS with preserved LVEF, seen in patients with small LV cavities (commonly in elderly women with chronic hypertension), severe diastolic dysfunction, atrial fibrillation, significant mitral and tricuspid valvular disease, pulmonary hypertension, right ventricular dysfunction, and cardiac amyloidosis (CA); and (3) normal-flow (SVi > 35 mL/m^2), low-gradient AS, explained by several factors, including a decreased flow rate despite a normal SVi, bradycardia, and/or abnormal arterial hemodynamics (systemic hypertension with prolonged ejection time).[10,12]

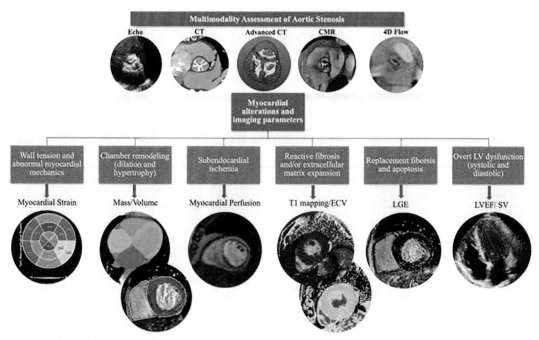

Fig. 1. Multimodality assessment of aortic stenosis: Beyond the valve. CMR, cardiac magnetic resonance; CT, computed tomography; ECV, extracellular volume; LGE, late gadolinium enhancement; LVEF, left ventricular ejection fraction; SV, stroke volume.

In low-flow low-gradient (LF-LG) AS, additional imaging modalities should be considered to confirm AS severity and guide timing to AVR. The use of hybrid imaging for AVA calculation by combining LVOT area by 3D echocardiography or contrast-enhanced CT paired with Doppler velocities has been proposed.[12] The use of CT can lead to overestimation of effective AVA and should be used with caution, and a larger AVA (1.2 cm^2) is considered for severe AS definition. Low-dose Dobutamine stress echocardiography (DSE) may be used to distinguish severe from pseudo-severe in patients with classical LF-LG AS; in true severe AS, there is an increased transaortic velocity and gradient with a fixed valve area after increasing SV greater than 20% with dobutamine. In those patients with inconclusive DSE (defined as failure to increase SV > 20%) and low-gradient AS with preserved LVEF, the aortic valve calcium score (an anatomic, load-independent measure) by CT has been suggested (Class 2a in recent guidelines).[4,12] An aortic valve calcification score greater than 1300 Agatston Units (AU) (420 AU/cm^2) in women or 2000 AU (527 AU/cm^2) in men is considered severe.[13]

The prognostic and clinical significance of the discordant LG-AS remains controversial, with some authors advocating for LG-AS as a severe and advanced form of AS associated with increased interstitial fibrosis, reduced LV longitudinal function, and poor prognosis, whereas others argue for being a less severe phenotype that can be safely monitored clinically. De Azevedo and colleagues, in their analysis of a large cohort (70% conservatively managed patients), confirmed that the survival of discordant LG-AS is better than that of HG-AS and worse than moderate AS patients. At comparable mean gradients, the lower the AVAi, the worse the prognosis, whereas at comparable AVAi, the higher the mean gradient, the worse the prognosis.[9]

Furthermore, in a cohort study including patients with paradoxical LG-AS, moderate AS, and HG-AS, Clavel and colleagues demonstrated that patients with paradoxical LG-AS have a worse prognosis than patients with moderate AS or HG-AS and benefit from AVR.[14] In a population of 1974 patients with moderate AS (AVA >1.0 and ≤ 1.5 cm^2), Stassen and colleagues demonstrated that the discordant patterns are frequent (40%), and LF-LG moderate AS may be associated with increased mortality compared with concordant moderate AS.[15]

Such conflicting data highlight the challenges in predicting future events in severe AS and probably depends on different underlying myocardial phenotypes. Therefore, a more comprehensive approach could guide the appropriate clinical decision-making, integrating symptoms, multiple

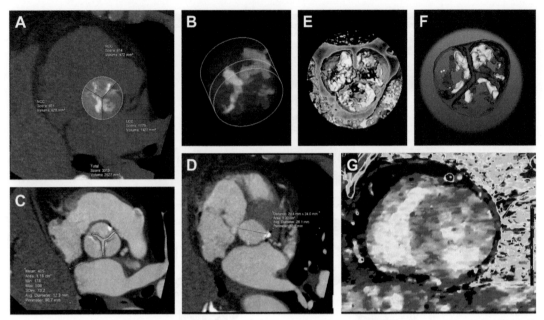

Fig. 2. Comprehensive AS characterization with CCT. (*A, B*) Aortic valve calcium quantification (*TeraRecon*). (*C, D*) AVA and left ventricular outflow tract (LVOT) planimetry. (*E*) VR of the aortic valve. (*F*) Virtual valve biopsy (*Autoplaque*). (*G*) Late iodine enhancement (Z effective image from *Intellispace Portal*).

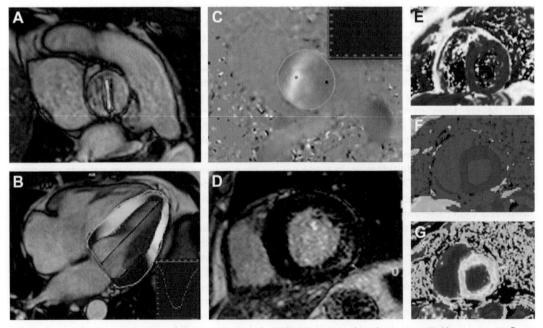

Fig. 3. Comprehensive evaluation of aortic stenosis with CMR. (*A*) Aortic valve planimetry. (*B*) Phase contrast flow and velocity assessment. (*C*) Feature tracking GLS. (*D*) Late gadolinium enhancement. (*E, F*) T2, T1 native, and (*G*) ECV mapping.

imaging modalities, and parameters to confirm the actual severity of the valve disease and the extent of myocardial damage caused by AS.

ASYMPTOMATIC SEVERE AORTIC STENOSIS AND THE MYOCARDIUM

Symptoms are often the primary driver for the initial evaluation and/or the reason for referral to cardiology; however, not uncommonly patients with severe AS are asymptomatic at the time of diagnosis.[16] AVR among asymptomatic severe AS patients has a class 1 recommendation for those with LV dysfunction or those undergoing other cardiac surgery and a class 2a recommendation for those with very severe AS or hemodynamic or exercise intolerance with exercise testing.[4] The optimal timing of follow-up and intervention in asymptomatic severe AS remains debated, more so with the exponential growth of transcatheter interventions. A recent systematic review and meta-analysis by Jaiswal and colleagues in asymptomatic severe AS reported that early surgical AVR ($n = 765$) was safer than conservative management ($n = 784$) in high-risk AS patients[17] specifically with lower all-cause mortality and sudden cardiac death. The RECOVERY trial randomized 145 patients with very severe asymptomatic AS (AVA 0.75 cm^2, mean gradient ≥ 50 mm Hg, peak velocity ≥ 4.5 m/s) and LVEF greater than 50% to an early surgical AVR versus a watchful-waiting strategy.[18] The primary outcome of operative mortality or cardiovascular mortality was significantly lower for early AVR [1% vs 6% ($P<.05$) at 4 years and 1% vs 26% ($P = .003$) at 8 years], mostly driven by cardiovascular mortality [1% vs 15% (HR 0.09, 95% CI 0.01–0.67, $P<.05$)]. Furthermore, in the AVATAR trial, early surgical AVR was compared with conservative therapy in 157 patients with asymptomatic guidelines-defined severe AS.[19] In an intention-to-treat analysis, patients randomized to early surgery had a significantly lower incidence of the primary composite end-point (HR 0.46 [95% CI, 0.23–0.90]; $P = .02$).

There are currently two ongoing multicenter, randomized controlled clinical trials focusing on outcomes of early AVR in the asymptomatic severe AS population. The EARLY transcatheter aortic valve replacement (TAVR) trial (NCT03042104) intends to investigate outcomes for asymptomatic severe AS patients with high surgical risk who undergo TAVR compared with a watchful waiting strategy. The EVOLVED study (NCT03094143) evaluates the use of biomarkers (high sensitivity (hs)-troponin), electrocardiogram (ECG), and

CMR to identify high-risk patients with asymptomatic severe AS and compare outcomes to those patients randomized to receive early AVR versus conservative medical management. These trials could help guide future practice and shape guideline-directed management in this asymptomatic severe AS population.

The outcomes observed from the RECOVERY and AVATAR trial highlight the risk associated with conservative management of asymptomatic severe AS and the need for closer follow-up and frequent reassessment for possible AVR despite LVEF greater than 50%. The use of additional imaging modalities such as CMR and GLS allows better identification of subclinical myocardial dysfunction, dyssynchrony, myocardial injury, and remodeling before the development of overt systolic dysfunction.[9,20]

One meta-analysis by Magne and colleagues investigating the significance of CMR-obtained LV GLS reported that among 1067 patients with asymptomatic severe AS (AVAi < 0.6 cm^2/m^2) and LVEF greater than 50% who did not undergo AVR, a GLS of less than 14.7% was associated with increased all-cause mortality (HR 3.58; 95% CI 1.84–6.99; $P<.0001$; $I^2 = 0$, $P<.0001$).[21] This suggests that compared with LVEF, LV GLS may be a better predictor of survival, thereby serving as a potential tool to guide AVR timing (Table 1).

Although impairment of LV GLS in severe AS is load-dependent, it has been associated with increased myocardial fibrosis.[21,22] LV fibrosis can be divided into two types (1) reactive interstitial fibrosis and (2) focal replacement fibrosis. Reactive interstitial fibrosis occurs in the early stages of AS; it can be identified using CMR native T1 mapping or extracellular volume (ECV) fraction derived from native and post-contrast T1 maps (see Fig. 2). These two parameters have been validated against histology and correlate with AS severity, LV mass, symptom status, and LV systolic function.[23,24] Moreover, the native T1 value was found to be an independent predictor of outcomes, in addition to other prognosticators such as EuroSCORE II or late gadolinium enhancement (LGE).[25] In 440 patients with severe AS undergoing AVR, Everett and colleagues demonstrated that ECV fraction was the strongest prognostic indicator, even superior to LVEF.[24] Importantly, interstitial fibrosis may be reversible following AVR.[6] On the other hand, replacement fibrosis in the context of AS represents a more advanced stage of the disease. The classic pattern of LGE uptake has been described as intramyocardial or "midwall." In a large study involving 674 patients

Table 1
Advanced myocardial imaging biomarkers in aortic stenosis

Echocardiography	CMR[5,6,24,53,54]	CCT
LV GLS[21,55] • Abnormal even when EF ≥ 50% • Strong prognostic value • > −14.7% was associated with a 2.5-fold increased risk of death LV myocardial work[56] • Myocardial deformation + LV afterload • Associated with heart failure incidence	LGE • Present in 27%–51% • Associated with AS severity, LV systolic, and diastolic dysfunction • Predicts mortality. • Pattern: Subendocardial (ischemic) vs Mid-myocardial (nonischemic) • Replacement fibrosis (irreversible) Native T1 • Diffuse fibrosis • Correlated with collagen volume fraction • Increased with disease severity ECV $_{CMR}$ • ECV > 28% in up to 54% with severe AS • Predicts mortality • Interstitial fibrosis (reversible with AVR) T2 (edema/inflammation) FT-GLS • Associated with outcomes post-AVR Stress perfusion • Coronary epicardial disease • Microvascular ischemia	ECV$_{CT}$[57] • Correlated with ECV$_{CMR}$ and histology • Prognostic value in AS + TTR-amyloid pre-TAVR

Abbreviations: CCT, cardiovascular computed tomography; CMR, cardiovascular magnetic resonance; ECV, extracellular volume; FT, feature tracking; GLS, global longitudinal strain; LGE, late gadolinium enhancement; LV, left ventricle; TAVR, transcatheter aortic valve replacement; TTR, transthyretin.

with severe AS undergoing AVR, the presence and amount of LGE was a strong independent predictor of worse outcomes (every 1% increase in LGE mortality hazard ratio increased by 11% and cardiovascular mortality by 8%).[26]

Focusing on the left atrium (LA), Tan and colleagues sought to investigate the prognostic performance of LA strain in relation to clinical, echocardiographic variables and N-terminal-pro brain natriuretic peptide (NT-proBNP) in 173 patients with asymptomatic or minimally symptomatic severe AS with LVEF greater than 50%.[27] They found that LA strain parameters outperformed other key echocardiographic variables and NT-ProBNP in predicting clinical outcomes. In addition, in a similar asymptomatic severe AS cohort of 248 patients with LVEF≥50%, LA strain rate and AVA correlated to the presence of HF with preserved EF.[28]

The above-mentioned data show the extensive recent progress in the subclinical impact of

severe AS and the role of several biomarkers that allow early recognition of those high-risk patients who may benefit from prompt intervention.

EFFECTS OF MODERATE AORTIC STENOSIS ON THE MYOCARDIUM

Current guidelines do not recommend AVR for isolated moderate AS unless cardiac surgery is considered for another indication.[4] Nonetheless, the severity of AS and LV systolic function are continuous variables, and structural repercussions in the LV myocardium can occur in parallel with a progressive increase in AS severity. In patients with HF with reduced ejection fraction (HFrEF), the simultaneous presence of moderate AS may further hamper LV systolic function by increasing afterload. In a recent meta-analysis, by Coisne and colleagues,[29] among a total of 25 studies (12,143 moderate AS patients, 3.7 years of follow-up), pooled rates per 100 person-years were 9.0 (95% CI: 6.9–11.7) for all-cause death. The investigators depicted that moderate AS seems to be associated with a mortality risk higher than no or mild AS but lower than severe AS, which increases in specific population subsets.

Before reaching the stage of overt LV dysfunction, through the use of CMR, several studies have demonstrated the presence and prognostic implications of nonischemic myocardial fibrosis in patients with moderate or severe AS.[30] In 143 patients with moderate (40%) and severe AS, Dweck and colleagues showed that 38% had mid-wall LGE uptake patterns and was an independent predictor of mortality regardless of the presence of concomitant ischemic subendocardial scar.[26] Interestingly, in that study, more than one-half of the patients with mid-wall fibrosis who died had only moderate AS, and they would not have been considered for AVR under standard-of-care practice.

It has been shown that an LVEF ≥50% often already represents subclinical myocardial dysfunction and a value < 60% in the presence of moderate AS could be considered abnormal.[31] In moderate AS, LV GLS may have an additional value in assessing early myocardial dysfunction. In 287 patients with moderate AS and LVEF ≥50%, Zhu and colleagues showed that patients with more impaired LV GLS (>–15.2%) had higher mortality rates ($P <$ .001).[32] These findings were consistent among patients with LVEF ≥60% and those who underwent AVR. Moreover, Stassen and colleagues found that patients with moderate AS and preserved LVEF, but impaired LV GLS (>−16%) had equally worse outcomes than patients with reduced LVEF.[33] Similarly to severe AS, the concept of "cardiac damage" has been evaluated recently in 1245 patients with moderate AS and significantly higher mortality was found with increasing extent of abnormalities.[34]

Along with imaging parameters of LV remodeling, specific myocardial biomarkers may alert of an ongoing maladaptive response to pressure overload. For example, in 261 patients with moderate AS, higher levels of NT-proBNP were associated with increased mortality rates, even after adjusting for age, gender, comorbidities, and echocardiographic LV parameters.[35]

Evidence continues to accumulate (Table 2), supporting the notion of AS severity as a continuous variable, with increasing AS severity imposing an increased pressure load on the LV. Ongoing randomized trials may likely answer whether an earlier AVR may improve outcomes in selected patients with moderate AS. The TAVR UNLOAD trial (NCT02661451) aims to investigate the effect of mechanical unloading with TAVR in patients with symptomatic moderate AS and LVEF less than 50%. The PROGRESS trial (NCT04889872) will include patients ≥65 year old and moderate AS with cardiac dysfunction or symptoms to evaluate the benefit of optimal medical therapy (OMT) plus transfemoral TAVR versus OMT alone. Finally, the EXPAND II trial (NCT05149755) will compare OMT with TAVR in patients with symptomatic moderate AS and one of the following: one heart failure decompensation episode in the past year, elevated NT-proBNP levels, reduced GLS or E/e' over 14.

AORTIC STENOSIS AND CARDIAC AMYLOIDOSIS

CA is characterized by an extracellular deposit of amyloid fibrils within the myocardium and other cardiac structures; it shares several common features with AS, with a worse prognosis.[36] Overall, transthyretin (TTR) is the most prevalent type of CA associated with AS, especially in men aged greater than 70 years.[37] LV myocardial infiltration by amyloid fibrils causes increased biventricular wall thickness and stiffness, impairing LV diastolic and longitudinal systolic function and leading to restrictive cardiomyopathy.[38] Diastolic HF with preserved LVEF is the most common presentation, but nearly one-third of patients may have HFrEF.[39] These features are also common in patients with severe AS, which may mask the presence of a concomitant CA. In addition, aortic valve infiltration by amyloid may contribute to the initiation and progression of AS.[40] Limited data are available on CA prevalence either isolated or associated with AS. A recent study discovered CA in 11.8% of AS patients through bone scintigraphy and exclusion of light chain (AL)-CA.[41]

Until now, there has been no recommendation or consensus on whether patients with AS should be systematically screened for CA. The TTR-CA screening and diagnosis protocol is similar in AS and the general population, but it is more challenging because AS and CA share several features. In patients with AS, which raise "Red Flags" for suspicion of CA, it should be tested. TTE features such as a mitral annulus S' velocity ≤6 cm/s are useful in screening for CA in patients with AS and preserved LVEF.[42] LV GLS is often markedly reduced and preserved at the apex in CA, but the apical sparing may also be observed in patients with AS and no CA.[43] A paradoxical (preserved LVEF) LF-LG AS pattern should also raise suspicion for CA.[42]

Table 2
Summary of literature involving moderate aortic stenosis

Study	Type	Population	Female sex	Moderate as	Follow-up	Primary Endpoint	Results
Van Gils et al,[58] 2017	Retrospective multicenter	305 patients with moderate AS and LVEF<50%	25%	305	4 y	All-cause death, AVR, and HFH	• Primary endpoint in 61% • Male sex, NYHA III/IV, and Vmax were independent predictors
Strange et al,[59] 2019	Registry: National Echocardiographic Database of Australia (NEDA)	241,303 individuals with full spectrum of AS.	37% (of mod AS patients)	3315	5 y	All-cause death and CV mortality	• Primary end point in 56% of moderate AS and 67% in severe AS • Markedly increased risk (adjusted for age, sex, LVEF, and so forth) with AV mean gradient ≧20 mm Hg or Vmax≧3 m/s
Dweck et al,[26] 2011	Prospective registry	143 patients with CMR	33%	57(40%)	2 y	All-cause mortality	• Mid-wall fibrosis/LGE is an independent predictor of the primary endpoint (HR: 5.35; 95% CI: 1.16–24.56) • 50% of patients with mid-wall LGE had moderate AS • 50% of mid-wall LGE patients who died had moderate AS

Study	Design	Population	%	N	Follow-up	Endpoint	Key findings
Zhu et al,[32] 2020	Retrospective	287 patients with moderate AS and LVEF≥ 50%	53%	287	3.9 y	All-cause mortality	• Primary end point in 36% • GLS > −15.2% had higher mortality (HR 2.62 [95% CI 1.69–4.06]), even in those with LVEF≥60% and those undergoing AVR
Stassen et al,[60] 2022	Muti-registry data	1931 patients	48%	1931	3 y	All-cause mortality	• Concentric LVH in 36%. • LVH independently associated with mortality (HR 1.25 [95% CI 1.01–1.55])
Ito et al,[35] 2020	Retrospective	261 patients with moderate AS	36%	261	2.7 y	All-cause mortality	• Primary end point in 52% • NT-proBNP >888 pg/dL had higher mortality • Higher NT-pro BNP associated with higher mortality rate (HR 3.11 [95% CI 1.78–5.46]), even in those undergoing AVR

Abbreviations: AS, aortic stenosis; AVR, aortic valve replacement; CI, confidence interval; GLS, global longitudinal strain; HFH, heart failure hospitalization; HR, hazard ratio; LGE, late gadolinium enhancement; LVEF, left ventricular ejection fraction; LVH, left ventricular hypertrophy; NT-proBNP, N-terminal-pro brain natriuretic peptide; NYHA, New York Heart Association.

Table 3
Red flags imaging criteria to suspect and confirm cardiac amyloidosis in patients with aortic stenosis

Demographics	Elderly ≥ 65 y, Male Sex, African Descendant
Clinical features	HFpEF, RV failure (ascites, edema), disproportionate HF symptoms, conduction abnormalities, unilateral/bilateral carpal tunnel syndrome, deafness, lumbar spinal stenosis
Biomarkers	Chronic troponin ↑ without significant coronary artery disease (CAD)/chronic kidney disease (CKD), NT-proBNP/BNP ↑ disproportionate to AS severity in the absence of renal failure
ECG	Discordant low-voltage and LV wall thickness, pseudo-infarction pattern (Q waves) without history of myocardial infarction
Echocardiography	LV wall thickening (≥15 mm) disproportionate to AS severity Myocardial granular sparkling Severe LV concentric remodeling (RWT >0.5) Severity of LV diastolic dysfunction (Grade ≥2; E/e′>15) disproportionate to LVH Severe LV longitudinal systolic dysfunction with apical sparing LV global longitudinal strain ≥ −12% and/or apex/basal longitudinal strain ratio >2 Moderate/severe pulmonary hypertension Mitral S′ ≤6 cm/s RV wall hypertrophy (≥5 mm) Biatrial dilatation Atrial septal thickening Atrioventricular valve thickening (>2 mm)
CMR	Elevated native T1 mapping and extracellular volume Abnormal gadolinium kinetics with short T1 inversion scout sequences Circumferential and extensive late gadolinium enhancement (subendocardial, basal predominance)
Diagnostic confirmation	Serum/urine monoclonal free light chain protein (for AL-CA) Additional tissue biopsy offten required Bone scintigraphy (for TTR-CA). Histology on endomyocardial and/or extracardiac biopsies.

Abbreviations: AS, aortic stenosis; BNP, brain natriuretic peptide; CA, cardiac amyloidosis; CMR, cardiac magnetic resonance; ECG, electrocardiogram; HFpEF, heart failure with preserved ejection fraction; LV, left ventricular; NT-proBNP, N-terminal pro-brain natriuretic peptide; TTR-CA, transthyretin cardiac amyloidosis.

The high prevalence of low-flow state in patients with CA may be explained by severe concentric LV and LA remodeling, impairment of diastolic filling, markedly reduced LV longitudinal systolic function, and RV remodeling and dysfunction.[44] In patients with CA, DSE often fails to increase LV outflow significantly and thus provides inconclusive results. Hence, quantifying AV calcium burden using non-contrast CT appears to be the most appropriate imaging modality to confirm AS severity in patients with CA.[45]

Diagnostic features by CMR (Table 3) offer the possibility of differentiating CA from other cardiomyopathies associated with LV hypertrophy. Still, 15% of CMR examinations may be normal in patients with CA.[38] In the past decade,

CT has gained attention as a potential tool to assess ECV, a marker of myocardial fibrosis that increases moderately with diffuse fibrosis but massively with CA. Kidoh and colleagues[46] described the sensitivity of ECV for detecting CA in CT TAVR as 90% and a specificity of 92% (Fig. 4). ECV CT can reliably detect dual AS-amyloid pathology with only 3 min on top of the standard CT imaging evaluation and a small radiation burden (∼2.3 mSv).[46] The measured ECV CT does not just help detect but to track the degree of infiltration. Commonly used in the pre-TAVR evaluation, cardiac CT offers a possible one-stop-shop analysis of valvular morphology, AS severity, cardiac function, and myocardial characterization. Recently, CT-GLS was demonstrated feasible to detect subclinical

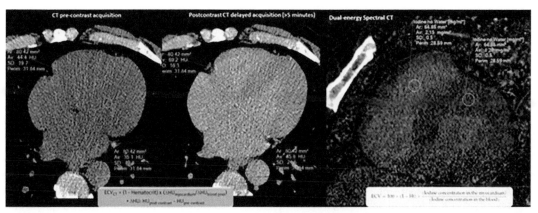

Fig. 4. CT evaluation of myocardial extracellular volume with conventional single energy scanner. Measurements were performed with *Philips Intellispace Portal v12.0*. CT evaluation of myocardial extracellular volume using dual-layer Spectral CT. Only one acquisition is required (delayed >5 minutes post-contrast) to obtain the iodine concentration of myocardium and blood poll. Images were acquired using *Philips IQon 64* scanner and analyzed with Philips Intellispace Portal v12.0.

myocardial changes in AS with a moderate correlation between CT-GLS and TTE (r = 0.62, P<.001).[47]

The clinical impact of myocardial amyloid deposition in patients with AS remains unclear. Further studies are needed to determine the optimal approaches for the screening and treatment of CA in patients with AS. Finally, specific guidelines should be developed to guide the heart team in deciding the type and the timing of treatment in symptomatic patients with severe AS and concomitant CA.

UTILIZATION OF FLUORODEOXYGLUCOSE PET IN EVALUATION OF AORTIC STENOSIS

Fluoro-2-deoxyglucose PET (FDG-PET) imaging can provide metabolic and functional assessment in evaluating AS and its effect on the myocardium. An increased glycolytic metabolic activity represents aortic valve inflammatory cell activity. Dweck and colleagues[48] demonstrated increased 18F-FDG uptake in hypermetabolic or inflamed tissues, and 18F-sodium fluoride (NaF) activity (a marker for active calcification) was noted to be greater than FDG activity in advanced AS.[49] Understanding that AS is an active local inflammatory condition not limited to the aortic valve, PET can provide an alternative method to evaluate the disease progression, risk stratification, and guide therapy in patients with AS.

In addition, as demonstrated by Zhou and colleagues, myocardial evaluation is also possible. Their work indicated that myocardial flow reserve (MFR) and stress myocardial blood flow were associated with adverse LV characteristics,

myocardial injury, and increased wall stress in AS.[50] MFR improved after AVR, suggesting that it may be an early marker for myocardial decompensation, likely due to the increased pressure gradient and wall stress leading to subendocardial ischemia and compounded by inherent microvascular dysfunction from common comorbidities, such as hypertension, CAD, and diabetes. Furthermore, PET could help differentiate between mimickers of LV remodeling secondary to AS, especially through the hybrid PET-MR approach that would allow characterization of LV volumes, mass, EF, and LGE burden.[51]

FUTURE PERSPECTIVES

Cardiac damage staging by echocardiography can predict both post-AVR outcomes and reverse remodeling beyond valve characteristics.[52] Although the valve is the primary insult, its interplay with the left ventricular myocardial response can manifest maladaptive changes earlier and ultimately determine the patient's prognosis and adaptive capabilities. Consequently, decisions regarding intervention, including timing and patient selection, should contemplate the myocardial response. New multimodality imaging tools, such as strain, parametric mapping, and LGE, present further opportunities to provide cardiac staging as a continuum. Of particular interest is the ability to identify the critical transition from adaptive, potentially reversible myocardial remodeling to maladaptive and potentially irreversible remodeling. Advanced imaging tools have unique capabilities to predict adverse myocardial remodeling and therefore refine timing for intervention in these patients, but they are still largely under-utilized, likely due to limited availability, standardization, and prospective validation. New trials are needed to investigate whether an imaging-guided earlier AVR approach may improve outcomes in patients with severe and moderate AS.

CLINICS CARE POINTS

- Accurate assessment of aortic stenosis severity is crucial for optimal management and timing of aortic valve replacement (AVR).
- Cardiac damage staging by echocardiography can predict both post-AVR outcomes and reverse remodeling beyond valve characteristics.
- New multimodality imaging tools, such as strain, parametric mapping, and LGE, present further opportunities to provide cardiac staging as a continuum.

DISCLOSURE

P Pina and D Lorenzatti are supported by grants from Amgen, United States and Philips, Netherlands. L Slipczuk has received an honorarium from Amgen, BMS, and Philips and grant support from Amgen and Philips. P Parwani is a consultant for Medtronic and Astrazeneca.

REFERENCES

1. Boskovski MT, Gleason TG. Current Therapeutic Options in Aortic Stenosis. Circ Res 2021;128(9):1398–417.
2. Choi YJ, Son JW, Kim EK, et al. Epidemiologic Profile of Patients With Valvular Heart Disease in Korea: A Nationwide Hospital-Based Registry Study. J Cardiovasc Imaging 2023;31(1):51–61.
3. Yadgir S, Johnson CO, Aboyans V, et al. Global, Regional, and National Burden of Calcific Aortic Valve and Degenerative Mitral Valve Diseases, 1990-2017. Circulation 2020;141(21):1670–80.
4. Otto CM, Nishimura RA, Bonow RO, et al. 2020 ACC/AHA Guideline for the Management of Patients With Valvular Heart Disease: Executive Summary: A Report of the American College of Cardiology/American Heart Association Joint Committee on Clinical Practice Guidelines. Circulation 2021;143(5):e35–71.
5. Ajmone Marsan N, Delgado V, Shah DJ, et al. Valvular heart disease: shifting the focus to the myocardium. Eur Heart J 2023;44(1):28–40.
6. Treibel TA, Kozor R, Schofield R, et al. Reverse Myocardial Remodeling Following Valve Replacement in Patients With Aortic Stenosis. J Am Coll Cardiol 2018;71(8):860–71.
7. Généreux P, Pibarot P, Redfors B, et al. Staging classification of aortic stenosis based on the extent of cardiac damage. Eur Heart J 2017;38(45):3351–8.
8. Bing R, Cavalcante JL, Everett RJ, et al. Imaging and Impact of Myocardial Fibrosis in Aortic Stenosis. JACC Cardiovasc Imaging 2019;12(2):283–96.
9. De Azevedo D, Tribouilloy C, Maréchaux S, et al. Prognostic Implications of Discordant Low-Gradient Severe Aortic Stenosis: Comprehensive Analysis of a Large Multicenter Registry. JACC Adv 2023;2(2):100254.
10. Guzzetti E, Annabi MS, Pibarot P, et al. Multimodality Imaging for Discordant Low-Gradient Aortic Stenosis: Assessing the Valve and the Myocardium. Front Cardiovasc Med 2020;7. Available at: https://www.frontiersin.org/articles/10.3389/fcvm.2020.570689. Accessed May 9, 2023.
11. Niederberger J, Schima H, Maurer G, et al. Importance of Pressure Recovery for the Assessment of Aortic Stenosis by Doppler Ultrasound. Circulation 1996;94(8):1934–40.
12. Delgado V, Clavel MA, Hahn RT, et al. How Do We Reconcile Echocardiography, Computed Tomography, and Hybrid Imaging in Assessing Discordant Grading of Aortic Stenosis Severity? JACC Cardiovasc Imaging 2019;12(2):267–82.
13. Pawade T, Sheth T, Guzzetti E, et al. Why and How to Measure Aortic Valve Calcification in Patients With Aortic Stenosis. JACC Cardiovasc Imaging 2019;12(9):1835–48.
14. Clavel MA, Dumesnil JG, Capoulade R, et al. Outcome of patients with aortic stenosis, small valve area, and low-flow, low-gradient despite preserved left ventricular ejection fraction. J Am Coll Cardiol 2012;60(14):1259–67.
15. Stassen J, Ewe SH, Singh GK, et al. Prevalence and Prognostic Implications of Discordant Grading and Flow-Gradient Patterns in Moderate Aortic Stenosis. J Am Coll Cardiol 2022;80(7):666–76.
16. Lindman BR, Clavel MA, Mathieu P, et al. Calcific aortic stenosis. Nat Rev Dis Primer 2016;2:16006.
17. Jaiswal V, Khan N, Jaiswal A, et al. Early surgery vs conservative management among asymptomatic aortic stenosis: A systematic review and meta-analysis. Int J Cardiol Heart Vasc 2022;43:101125.
18. Kang DH, Park SJ, Lee SA, et al. Early Surgery or Conservative Care for Asymptomatic Aortic Stenosis. N Engl J Med 2020;382(2):111–9.
19. Banovic M, Putnik S, Penicka M, et al. Aortic Valve Replacement Versus Conservative Treatment in Asymptomatic Severe Aortic Stenosis: The AVATAR Trial. Circulation 2022;145(9):648–58.

20. Lancellotti P, Donal E, Magne J, et al. Impact of global left ventricular afterload on left ventricular function in asymptomatic severe aortic stenosis: a two-dimensional speckle-tracking study. Eur J Echocardiogr J Work Group Echocardiogr Eur Soc Cardiol 2010;11(6):537–43.

21. Magne J, Cosyns B, Popescu BA, et al. Distribution and Prognostic Significance of Left Ventricular Global Longitudinal Strain in Asymptomatic Significant Aortic Stenosis: An Individual Participant Data Meta-Analysis. JACC Cardiovasc Imaging 2019; 12(1):84–92.

22. Kostakou PM, Tryfou ES, Kostopoulos VS, et al. Segmentally impaired left ventricular longitudinal strain: a new predictive diagnostic parameter for asymptomatic patients with severe aortic stenosis and preserved ejection fraction. Perfusion 2022; 37(4):402–9.

23. Chin CWL, Everett RJ, Kwiecinski J, et al. Myocardial Fibrosis and Cardiac Decompensation in Aortic Stenosis. JACC Cardiovasc Imaging 2017;10(11): 1320–33.

24. Everett RJ, Treibel TA, Fukui M, et al. Extracellular Myocardial Volume in Patients With Aortic Stenosis. J Am Coll Cardiol 2020;75(3):304–16.

25. Lee JM, Choi KH, Koo BK, et al. Prognostic Implications of Plaque Characteristics and Stenosis Severity in Patients With Coronary Artery Disease. J Am Coll Cardiol 2019;73(19):2413–24.

26. Dweck MR, Joshi S, Murigu T, et al. Midwall fibrosis is an independent predictor of mortality in patients with aortic stenosis. J Am Coll Cardiol 2011;58(12): 1271–9.

27. Tan ESJ, Jin X, Oon YY, et al. Prognostic Value of Left Atrial Strain in Aortic Stenosis: A Competing Risk Analysis. J Am Soc Echocardiogr Off Publ Am Soc Echocardiogr 2023;36(1):29–37.e5.

28. Mateescu AD, Călin A, Beladan CC, et al. Left Atrial Dysfunction as an Independent Correlate of Heart Failure Symptoms in Patients With Severe Aortic Stenosis and Preserved Left Ventricular Ejection Fraction. J Am Soc Echocardiogr Off Publ Am Soc Echocardiogr 2019;32(2):257–66.

29. Coisne A, Scotti A, Latib A, et al. Impact of Moderate Aortic Stenosis on Long-Term Clinical Outcomes. JACC Cardiovasc Interv 2022;15(16):1664–74.

30. Stassen J, Ewe SH, Pio SM, et al. Managing Patients With Moderate Aortic Stenosis. JACC Cardiovasc Imaging 2023. https://doi.org/10.1016/j.jcmg.2022.12.013.

31. Ito S, Miranda WR, Nkomo VT, et al. Reduced Left Ventricular Ejection Fraction in Patients With Aortic Stenosis. J Am Coll Cardiol 2018;71(12):1313–21.

32. Zhu D, Ito S, Miranda WR, et al. Left Ventricular Global Longitudinal Strain Is Associated With Long-Term Outcomes in Moderate Aortic Stenosis. Circ Cardiovasc Imaging 2020;13(4):e009958.

33. Stassen J, Pio SM, Ewe SH, et al. Left Ventricular Global Longitudinal Strain in Patients with Moderate Aortic Stenosis. J Am Soc Echocardiogr Off Publ Am Soc Echocardiogr 2022;35(8):791–800.e4.

34. Amanullah MR, Pio SM, Ng ACT, et al. Prognostic Implications of Associated Cardiac Abnormalities Detected on Echocardiography in Patients With Moderate Aortic Stenosis. JACC Cardiovasc Imaging 2021;14(9):1724–37.

35. Ito S, Miranda WR, Jaffe AS, et al. Prognostic Value of N-Terminal Pro-form B-Type Natriuretic Peptide in Patients With Moderate Aortic Stenosis. Am J Cardiol 2020;125(10):1566–70.

36. d'Humières T, Fard D, Damy T, et al. Outcome of patients with cardiac amyloidosis admitted to an intensive care unit for acute heart failure. Arch Cardiovasc Dis 2018;111(10):582–90.

37. Ruberg FL, Grogan M, Hanna M, et al. Transthyretin Amyloid Cardiomyopathy: JACC State-of-the-Art Review. J Am Coll Cardiol 2019;73(22):2872–91.

38. Ternacle J, Krapf L, Mohty D, et al. Aortic Stenosis and Cardiac Amyloidosis: JACC Review Topic of the Week. J Am Coll Cardiol 2019;74(21):2638–51.

39. González-López E, Gallego-Delgado M, Guzzo-Merello G, et al. Wild-type transthyretin amyloidosis as a cause of heart failure with preserved ejection fraction. Eur Heart J 2015;36(38):2585–94.

40. Audet A, Côté N, Couture C, et al. Amyloid substance within stenotic aortic valves promotes mineralization. Histopathology 2012;61(4):610–9.

41. Nitsche C, Scully PR, Patel KP, et al. Prevalence and Outcomes of Concomitant Aortic Stenosis and Cardiac Amyloidosis. J Am Coll Cardiol 2021;77(2): 128–39.

42. Castaño A, Narotsky DL, Hamid N, et al. Unveiling transthyretin cardiac amyloidosis and its predictors among elderly patients with severe aortic stenosis undergoing transcatheter aortic valve replacement. Eur Heart J 2017;38(38):2879–87.

43. Abecasis J, Lopes P, Santos RR, et al. Prevalence and significance of relative apical sparing in aortic stenosis: insights from an echo and cardiovascular magnetic resonance study of patients referred for surgical aortic valve replacement. Eur Heart J - Cardiovasc Imaging 2023. https://doi.org/10.1093/ehjci/jead032. jead032.

44. Galat A, Guellich A, Bodez D, et al. Aortic stenosis and transthyretin cardiac amyloidosis: the chicken or the egg? Eur Heart J 2016;37(47):3525–31.

45. Treibel TA, Fontana M, Gilbertson JA, et al. Occult Transthyretin Cardiac Amyloid in Severe Calcific Aortic Stenosis: Prevalence and Prognosis in Patients Undergoing Surgical Aortic Valve Replacement. Circ Cardiovasc Imaging 2016;9(8):e005066.

46. Kidoh M, Oda S, Takashio S, et al. CT Extracellular Volume Fraction versus Myocardium-to-Lumen Signal Ratio for Cardiac Amyloidosis. Radiology 2022. https://doi.org/10.1148/radiol.220542.

47. Fukui M, Xu J, Abdelkarim I, et al. Global longitudinal strain assessment by computed tomography in severe aortic stenosis patients - Feasibility using feature tracking analysis. J Cardiovasc Comput Tomogr 2019;13(2):157–62.

48. Dweck MR, Jones C, Joshi NV, et al. Assessment of valvular calcification and inflammation by positron emission tomography in patients with aortic stenosis. Circulation 2012;125(1):76–86.

49. Marincheva-Savcheva G, Subramanian S, Qadir S, et al. Imaging of the aortic valve using fluorodeoxyglucose positron emission tomography increased valvular fluorodeoxyglucose uptake in aortic stenosis. J Am Coll Cardiol 2011;57(25):2507–15.

50. Zhou W, Sun YP, Divakaran S, et al. Association of Myocardial Blood Flow Reserve With Adverse Left Ventricular Remodeling in Patients With Aortic Stenosis: The Microvascular Disease in Aortic Stenosis (MIDAS) Study. JAMA Cardiol 2022;7(1):93–9.

51. Nordström J, Kvernby S, Kero T, et al. Left-ventricular volumes and ejection fraction from cardiac ECG-gated 15O-water positron emission tomography compared to cardiac magnetic resonance imaging using simultaneous hybrid PET/MR. J Nucl Cardiol 2022. https://doi.org/10.1007/s12350-022-03154-7.

52. Parikh PB. Predicting Futility in Aortic Stenosis: What's the Holdup? J Am Coll Cardiol 2022;80(8):801–3.

53. Lee SP, Lee W, Lee JM, et al. Assessment of diffuse myocardial fibrosis by using MR imaging in asymptomatic patients with aortic stenosis. Radiology 2015;274(2):359–69.

54. Fukui M, Annabi MS, Rosa VEE, et al. Comprehensive myocardial characterization using cardiac magnetic resonance associates with outcomes in low gradient severe aortic stenosis. Eur Heart J Cardiovasc Imaging 2022;24(1):46–58.

55. Thellier N, Altes A, Appert L, et al. Prognostic Importance of Left Ventricular Global Longitudinal Strain in Patients with Severe Aortic Stenosis and Preserved Ejection Fraction. J Am Soc Echocardiogr Off Publ Am Soc Echocardiogr 2020;33(12):1454–64.

56. Fortuni F, Butcher SC, van der Kley F, et al. Left Ventricular Myocardial Work in Patients with Severe Aortic Stenosis. J Am Soc Echocardiogr Off Publ Am Soc Echocardiogr 2021;34(3):257–66.

57. Treibel TA, Patel KP, Cavalcante JL. Extracellular Volume Imaging in Aortic Stenosis During Routine Pre-TAVR Cardiac Computed Tomography. JACC Cardiovasc Imaging 2020;13(12):2602–4.

58. van Gils L, Clavel MA, Vollema EM, et al. Prognostic Implications of Moderate Aortic Stenosis in Patients With Left Ventricular Systolic Dysfunction. J Am Coll Cardiol 2017;69(19):2383–92.

59. Strange G, Stewart S, Celermajer D, et al. Poor Long-Term Survival in Patients With Moderate Aortic Stenosis. J Am Coll Cardiol 2019;74(15):1851–63.

60. Stassen J, Ewe SH, Hirasawa K, et al. Left ventricular remodelling patterns in patients with moderate aortic stenosis. Eur Heart J Cardiovasc Imaging 2022;23(10):1326–35.

Multimodality Imaging for the Assessment of Mitral Valve Disease

Dae-Hee Kim, MD, PhD

KEYWORDS

- Mitral valve • Echocardiography • Magnetic resonance imaging • Computed tomography

---

KEY POINTS

- The mitral valve complex's proper function needs the integrity of leaflets, annulus, chordae, papillary muscles, ventricle, and atrium. Functional, structural, or geometric distortion of one or more of these parts may cause valvular dysfunction. Therefore, comprehensive evaluations of these parameters with any imaging modality are crucial.
- Echocardiography is the primary imaging modality for visualizing the mitral valve. Three-dimensional (3D) imaging provides incremental value in assessing the severity of valvular heart disease and establishing its mechanism. For patients undergoing transcatheter intervention, real-time 3D images facilitate manipulating the catheter, to position and orient the device.
- Roles of computed tomography and cardiac MRI (CMR) are increasing. The utility of CMR for the evaluation of mitral regurgitation has recently been adopted as part of the guideline.

INTRODUCTION

The burden of valvular heart disease is increases with age. Mitral valve (MV) disease is the most common valvular heart disease. The prevalence in subjects older than 75 years is almost 10%.[1] Imaging is needed to assess or be evaluated for (1) valve morphology to determine the etiology (anatomic assessment), (2) valve function and the severity of valvular heart disease (hemodynamic assessment), (3) remodeling of the left ventricle (LV) and right ventricle (RV), and (4) preplanning and guidance of percutaneous intervention. Echocardiography is the primary imaging modality for visualizing the MV. Although roles of computed tomography (CT) and cardiac magnetic resonance (CMR) are increasing, echocardiography serves as the first-line imaging modality for diagnosis and serial follow-up in most cases. This review summarizes the roles of multimodality imaging currently available from research fields to daily clinical practice.

NORMAL MITRAL VALVE ANATOMY

The MV apparatus comprises an annulus, 2 leaflets, chordae tendineae, and papillary muscles (Fig. 1).[2] The MV annulus, a D-shaped ring rather than circular shape positioned in the left atrioventricular groove, extends from 2 fibrous trigones located at either end of the area of fibrous continuity between the aortic leaflet of the MV and the aortic root.[3] This straight border forms the anterior part of the annulus, which is in fibrous continuity with the aortic valve. The remaining border of the annulus forms the posterior annulus. Annular remodeling occurs predominantly in the posterior part of the annulus (asymmetric annular dilation), because the posterior part of the annulus faces pliant endocardium, not a fibrous skeleton.[4]

This article originally appeared in *Cardiology Clinics*, Volume 39 Issue 2, May 2021.

Division of Cardiology, Asan Medical Center, College of Medicine, University of Ulsan, 388-1, Poongnap-dong, Songpa-ku, Seoul 138-736, Korea

E-mail address: daehee74@amc.seoul.kr

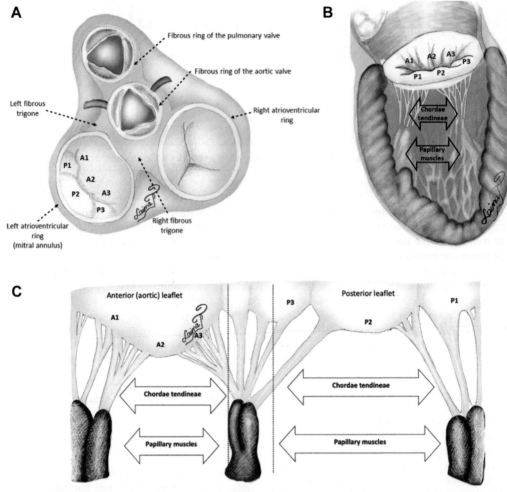

Fig. 1. Anatomy of the MV apparatus. Craniocaudal view of the heart (*A*) with components of the fibrous skeleton. Longitudinal cross-sectional view (*B*) highlighting the position of the MV, chordae tendineae and PMs. Expanded view of the MV leaflets, chordae, and proximal parts of the PMs (*C*). (Augustinas Tumenas, Laima Tamkeviciute, Reda Arzanauskiene, Monika Arzanauskaite, Multimodality Imaging of the Mitral Valve: Morphology, Function, and Disease, Current Problems in Diagnostic Radiology, 50 (6), 2021, 905-924, https://doi.org/10.1067/j.cpra-diol.2020.09.013.)

Anterior and posterior mitral leaflets are not equal in size.[5] The anterior leaflet attaches to one-third of the annulus but encloses a larger portion of the valve orifice than the posterior leaflet dose. The anterior leaflet is one of the parts of LV outflow tract (LVOT) during systole, causing outflow tract obstruction in hypertrophic obstructive cardiomyopathy.[6] Three segments form each leaflet: A1, A2, and A3 in the anterior leaflet and P1, P2, and P3 in the posterior leaflet. The clefts or indentations along the free margin of the posterior leaflet make it a scalloped appearance. Despite the absence of indentations, similar terminology is applied for the anterior leaflet scallops. Three scallops are not equal in size, and middle scallops are larger in most cases.[7] When the leaflets coapt during diastole,

the view of the valve from the atrium resembles a smile. Each end of the coaptation line is named as a commissure. Normally, the valvar leaflets are thin, translucent, and soft, and each leaflet has an atrial and a ventricular surface.

The MV leaflets are braced by chordae, and attach to 2 papillary muscles (PMs). The tendinous cords are stringlike structures that connect the ventricular surface or the free edge of the leaflets to the PMs.[8] The first-order cords are inserted into the free edge of the MV. Second-order cords insert on the ventricular surface of the leaflets beyond the free edge, forming the rough zone. Third-order cords are connected only to the mural leaflet because they arise directly from the ventricular wall.[8] The Toronto group classified them into leaflets and interleaflet

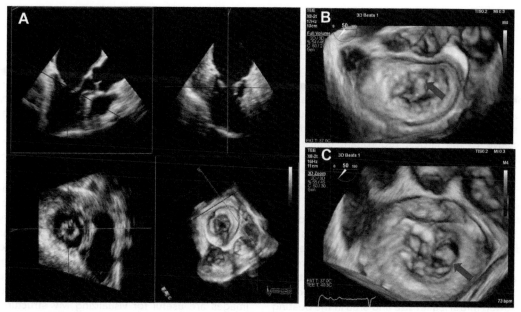

Fig. 2. Multiplanar reconstruction (MPR) mode on 3D TEE to assess the MV. Using MPR mode in patients with mitral stenosis allows a more accurate valve measurement (*A*). Three-dimensional reconstruction of the MV en face in an orientation identical to the surgeon's view shows A2 prolapse with ruptured chordae (*red arrow, B*). Three-dimensional en face view depicting a medical commissural prolapse (*red arrow, C*). Differentiation between commissural prolapse and A3, P3 prolapse is crucial in the era of the MV intervention.

or commissural cords.[9] Viewed from the atrial aspect, the 2 PMs are located below the commissures, positioning in anterolateral and posteromedial directions. The anterolateral PM is a single in 70% of cases, and the posteromedial PM is 2 or 3 in number or 1 PM with 2 or 3 heads in 60%.[8]

Echocardiography

Transthoracic echocardiography (TTE) is the first-line imaging modality for screening, assessment, diagnosis, and surveillance of valvular disease. For MV disease, TTE is still the mainstream for evaluating the etiology, anatomic morphology, and grade of mitral regurgitation (MR) or stenosis (MS). The proper function of the MV complex needs the integrity of leaflets, mitral annulus, chordae, PMs, LV, and left atrium (LA). Functional, structural, or geometric distortion of 1 or more of these parts may cause valvular dysfunction.[10] The grading of severity of valvular heart disease will not be discussed herein. Comprehensive approaches with multimodality imaging are especially required for the assessment of MR.[11]

Three-dimensional (3D) imaging provides incremental value in the assessment of severity of valvular stenosis (Fig. 2A) or regurgitation (Fig. 2B) and in establishing its mechanism. Traditionally, two-dimensional (2D) imaging requires

multiple view acquisitions, including modified views of the MV, to make a detailed assessment of MV morphology, adjuring longer study time and expert interpretation. Three-dimensional transesophageal echocardiography (TEE) has become widely used in operating rooms and cardiac catheterization laboratories. Three-dimensional TEE has been proven to be superior to 2D TEE in the assessment of both MV anatomy and MR.[12] One reason for this superiority is that 3D TEE allows the MV to be visualized en face in an orientation identical to the surgeon's view of the MV intraoperatively (Fig. 2B, C), and 3D TEE enables the person with relatively little training to acquire high-quality real-time 3D images even in a single beat. Three-dimensional echocardiography has multiple acquisition modes and display options (simultaneous multiplane imaging, tomographic slices, surface rendering, and volume rendering); moreover, simultaneous 2D multiplane imaging ("x-plane or biplane mode") in a modifiable angulation.[13] Accurate preoperative or preprocedural assessment of the valve anatomy and location of lesions are critical in the management of patients with severe MR.[14] This information determines whether the patient should undergo valve repair or replacement and influences the timing of surgery accordingly.

For patients undergoing transcatheter intervention for MR, adequate patient selection for these therapies requires a precise assessment of MV anatomy and function. Moreover, live 3D TEE en face views of the MV facilitate manipulation of the catheter, to position and orient the device without damaging adjacent structures (Fig. 3A, B). The biplane (x-plane) views show simultaneously the bi-commissural, and the 3-chamber long-axis planes (Fig. 3C) is most frequently used to fine-tune the orientation of the device relative to the largest regurgitant orifice area and perpendicular to the coaptation line.

Further anatomic or geometric qualifications with echocardiography

In patients with hypertrophic cardiomyopathy, LV outflow tract obstruction (LVOTO) is produced by systolic anterior motion of the MV. Clinical implications of MV size in hypertrophic cardiomyopathy have been elucidated with 2D and 3D echocardiography, which recently allowed mitral leaflet size and area in the beating heart (Fig. 4).[15,16] In vivo measurement of mitral leaflet area makes it possible to understand more on the mechanisms of ischemic/function MR in detail using 3D echocardiography.[4,17,18] Recently, commercialized software supports the measurement.[19,20]

The visualization of mitral annulus shape using 3D echocardiography has contributed to the development of nonplanar mitral annuloplasty rings.[21] Comprehensive analysis of annulus geometry, including area, perimeter, nonplanar angle, diameters, intertrigone distance, and height can provide valuable information to reveal the mechanism of valvular heart disease (Fig. 5).[22,23] Minimal mitral annulus dimensions are present in early systole, and annulus dimensions increase toward late systole. Changes in all parameters acquired from annulus geometry can be calculated during the cardiac cycle; annular dynamics differ between healthy subjects and patients with MV disease.[24]

Computed Tomography Scan

Cardiac CT scan acquires the images with the injection of contrast agents, and protocol is structured to allow assessment of the coronary arteries as well. The pathologic imaging findings of the MV including prolapse, vegetation, and coaptation gap, can be well demonstrated in the systolic phase of the cardiac cycle. Cine reconstruction methods using volume-rendered images are useful for visualizing MV structure. At our institution, cardiac CT for evaluation of both the coronary artery and MV is performed with a second-generation dual-source CT scanner (Definition Flash; Siemens, Erlangen, Germany). The images acquired in the mid-systolic phase are used to evaluate the MV. Images are reconstructed with the 5% R-R interval (20 images per 1 cardiac cycle) for retrospective electrocardiogram (ECG)-gated scanning and at 10-ms intervals for prospective ECG-triggered scanning.[25]

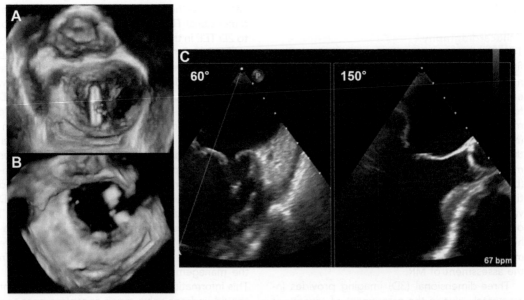

Fig. 3. Real-time 3D images make it possible to check a clip orientation during the percutaneous MV edge to edge repair (*A, B*). The clip is recommended to be placed perpendicular to the coaptation line. Reducing 3D gain can visualize the clip in the LV (*B*). X-plane imaging is advantageous to guide the percutaneous mitral intervention. The bi-commissural (*left*) and LVOT view (*right*) images are crucial for the MitraClip intervention (*C*).

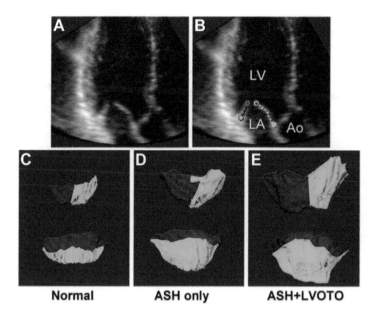

Fig. 4. Component view with mitral leaflet traces for 3D reconstruction (*A, B*). Representative open mitral leaflet area measurements in green and purple for anterior and posterior leaflets viewed from the side (*C* through *E*, top row, lateral commissure in foreground) and LVOT aspect below, largest in asymmetric septal hypertrophy (ASH) and ASH with LVOTO. Ao, aorta. (*From* Kim DH, Handschumacher MD, Levine RA, et al. In vivo measurement of mitral leaflet surface area and subvalvular geometry in patients with asymmetrical septal hypertrophy: insights into the mechanism of outflow tract obstruction. Circulation. 2010;122(13):1298-1307; with permission.)

Normal   **ASH only**   **ASH+LVOTO**

Assessment of prolapse segment with computed tomography scan

In our clinical practice, we review the quality of images with 4-dimensional multiphase CT data including the 3-chamber view. We found that the best-quality images were obtained during the 25% to 35% cardiac phases in approximately 80% of patients with MV prolapse.[25] A step-by-step method for the image reconstruction of MV can be summarized as follows: (1) determine the best cardiac phase; (2) identify the location and extent of disease on sagittal and coronal views of the MV by using a multiplanar reformatted technique (anterior vs posterior leaflet in the sagittal view; medial, middle, or lateral scallops in the coronal view); and (3) recheck the extent

and location of the disease on the 3D volume-rendered image (Fig. 6).[25]

The localization of the MV prolapse segment is feasible on a per-scallop basis, but it may underestimate the extent of prolapsed scallop compared with TEE, particularly in patients with multiple-scallop lesions. The per-scallop sensitivity of cardiac CT was slightly lower than that of echocardiography (80% vs 87%, $P = .004$), with similar specificity (both 95%).[26]

Detection of paravalvular leakage in patients with prosthetic heart valve

Paravalvular leakage (PVL) is defined as an abnormal communication between the sewing ring and valve annulus and the prevalence of

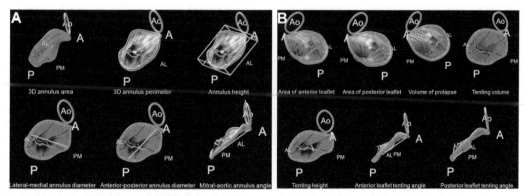

Fig. 5. Parameters for MV annulus geometry (*A*). Parameters for MV leaflet geometry (*B*). A, anterior; AL, antero-lateral; Ao, aortic annulus; P, posterior, PM, posteromedial. (*From* Song JM, Jung YJ, Jung YJ, et al. Three-dimensional remodeling of mitral valve in patients with significant regurgitation secondary to rheumatic versus prolapse etiology. Am J Cardiol. 2013;111(11):1631-1637; with permission.)

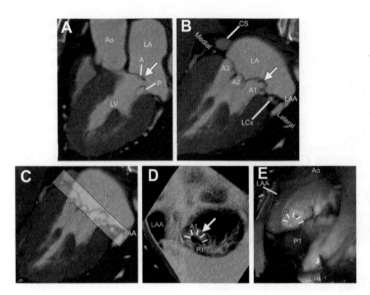

Fig. 6. Reconstruction of CT images of the MV to evaluate the extent and location of MV prolapse. A1, A2, and A3 = lateral, middle, and medial scallops of the anterior leaflet, respectively; P1, P2, and P3 = lateral, middle, and medial scallops of the posterior leaflet, respectively. Parasagittal reconstructed CT image shows MV prolapse in the A1 portion (A). A coronal reconstructed CT image shows a prolapsed scallop of the MV (arrow) near the left atrial appendage, which is a landmark of a lateral direction in the MV annulus. The proximal left circumflex artery (LCX) is also located in the lateral direction, and the coronary sinus (CS) and interatrial septum are located in the medial direction (B). Coronal thin-section maximum intensity projection reconstructed CT image obtained at the level of the valve shows the section thickness used to generate the surgeon's view (C). Surgeon's view of the MV obtained with thin-section (15-mm) volume rendering shows that the A1 scallop is prolapsed (D). Intraoperative photograph obtained with a robot-assisted surgery system shows that the locations of the prolapsed scallop and left atrial appendage (LAA) correspond with the CT findings (E). Ao, ascending aorta. (From Koo HJ, Yang DH, Oh SY, et al. Demonstration of mitral valve prolapse with CT for planning of mitral valve repair. Radiographics. 2014;34(6):1537-1552; with permission.)

PVL after MV replacement ranges from 3% to 15%.[27] For severe symptomatic PVL, surgical corrections perform either repair of the leak or re-replacement have been recommended. However, the recurrence rates range from 12% to 35%, and therefore percutaneous device closure has been introduced as an alternative option to treat PVL.[28] For decision making in PVL treatment, anatomic information, including the size, shape, and the 3D relationship with adjacent structures should be considered as parts of pre-procedural planning. Echocardiography is the primary modality of choice that provides excellent temporal resolution and real-time imaging capabilities with color Doppler information, but sometimes image quality can be compromised. In contrast, cardiac CT can give more precise anatomic details, including the exact location and morphology of the PVLs. Pretreatment planning could be better tailored and individualized with cardiac CT scan (Fig. 7).[29]

Detection and diagnosis of infective endocarditis

Echocardiography is the imaging method of choice for the diagnosis of infective endocarditis (IE), but the operator dependency and poor sonic window caused by calcifications or detection on vegetation on mechanical prosthetic valves are still limitations. A recent meta-analysis showed that CT might provide incremental value to TEE for

diagnosing prosthetic valve IE.[30] Kim and colleagues[31] reported the overall detection rate of vegetation was inferior in CT compared with TEE (97.3% vs 72.0%), but cardiac CT shows comparable diagnostic performance with TEE for large vegetation (≥10 mm). TEE was better for detecting small vegetation, valve perforation, and intracardiac fistula, whereas CT was more useful for detecting perivalvular abscess and coronary artery disease.[31] In contrast, another report showed similar sensitivities between CT and TEE to detect IE, and excellent interobserver agreement.[32]

Leaflet size, annulus geometry, and relationship with papillary muscles

Mitral leaflet area and annulus area measured by CT were comparable with 3D echocardiography, and there was no difference in agreement with 3D TEE for patients scanned with single-source versus dual-source CT.[33] Song and colleagues[34] explored geometric predictors of LVOTO in patients with hypertrophic cardiomyopathy by using cardiac CT and found that anterior mitral leaflet length and the distance between lateral PM base and LV apex were independent predictors of LVOTO. Cardiac CT has an advantage of more accurate evaluation of the 3D geometry of myocardial hypertrophy pattern and PMs than CMR and echocardiography.[29,32,34]

In the ear of transcatheter MV replacement (TMVR), CT is becoming a critical imaging

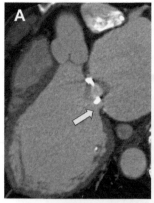
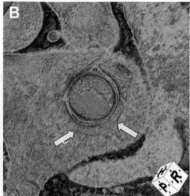
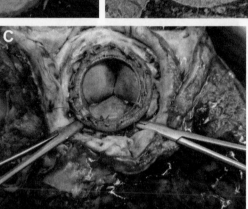

Fig. 7. Large crescent-shaped dehiscence (*yellow arrows*) that involved posterior part of the mitral annulus on CT images (*A, B*). A single large PVL in surgical inspection was confirmed. Surgical instruments indicate the medial and lateral ends of the paravalvular dehiscence (*C*).

modality for identifying the MV anatomy and its spatial relationships with other structures. The parameters measuring the MV annulus geometry are essential to select the size of transcatheter MV annuloplasty devices and TMVR. The assessment of MV annulus calcification is essential to check the feasibility of various transcatheter therapies.[10] For TMVR planning, truncation of the saddle-shaped annular contour at a virtual line connecting both trigones (trigone-to-trigone [TT] distance), has been used.[24] Three-dimensional segmentation and post-processing yield annular area and perimeter, TT distance, septal-to-lateral distance (A2-to-P2 distance, minor diameter), and the intercommissural (IC) distance (major diameter).[24] Similar post-processing using 3D echocardiography full-volume set can be performed off-line (Fig. 8).

CARDIAC MAGNETIC RESONANCE IMAGING

CMR provides a comprehensive evaluation of cardiac anatomy, function, and myocardial tissue characterization, and the usefulness to assess valvular heart disease, especially regurgitation,

is increasingly recognized. The utility of CMR for the evaluation of valvular regurgitation has recently been adopted as part of the joint American Society of Echocardiography and the Society of Cardiovascular Magnetic Resonance recommendations for the noninvasive evaluation of native valvular regurgitation.[11] For assessment of the severity of MR, CMR has become an established noninvasive imaging modality to assess the severity of MR (Fig. 9).[35]

Valve Structure and Ventricular Function Assessment

To visualize the morphology and motion of the MV from any desired image orientation, balanced steady-state free precession (SSFP) sequence cine imaging techniques have been widely used for the evaluation of valvular structures in motion, because it can provide a high signal-to-noise ratio (excellent contrast) between the blood pool and myocardium. Older sequences such as "black blood" turbo-spin-echo (TSE) techniques (T1-weighted and T2-weighted TSE imaging techniques) can be used for the evaluation of valvular masses such as vegetations or tumors.[36] Quantification of LV size

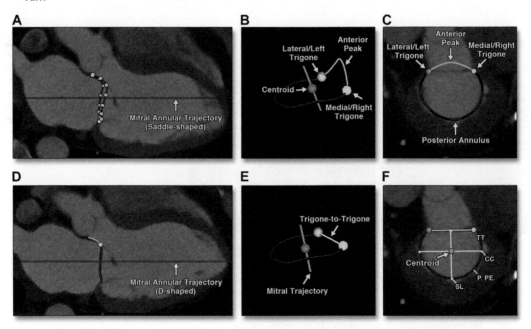

Fig. 8. Saddle-shaped annulus segmentation as a cubic spline interpolation (A). Pink line = anterior peak; red line = posterior peak (posterior mitral leaflet insertion, P. PE.); green and blue dots = fibrous trigones (B). Importantly, the anterior peak projects into the LVOT (short-axis view [C] and long-axis view [D]). The more planar D-shaped annular contour is created by truncating the saddle-shaped contour at the TT distance (yellow lines [E, F]). Important measurements are the projected area setal-to-lateral (SL) and intercommissural (CC) distances; the latter is oriented perpendicularly to SL while transecting through the centroid (F). (From Blanke P, Naoum C, Webb J, et al. Multimodality Imaging in the Context of Transcatheter Mitral Valve Replacement: Establishing Consensus Among Modalities and Disciplines. JACC Cardiovasc Imaging. 2015;8(10):1191-1208; with permission.)

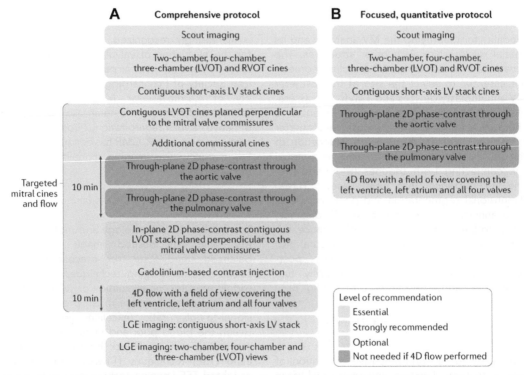

Fig. 9. Recommended cardiovascular MRI protocols for the assessment of MR. Comprehensive cardiovascular MRI protocol for the assessment of MR (A). Focused, quantitative protocol (B). LGE, late gadolinium enhancement; RVOT, right ventricular outflow tract. (From Garg P, Swift AJ, Zhong L, et al. Assessment of mitral valve regurgitation by cardiovascular magnetic resonance imaging. Nat Rev Cardiol. 2020;17(5):298-312; with permission.)

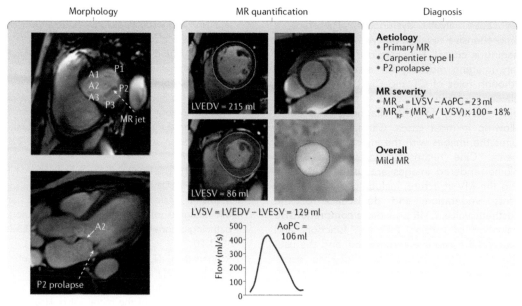

Fig. 10. MR assessment in a patient with ischemic cardiomyopathy. Incomplete coaptation owing to ventricular dilatation is seen on the short-axis cines (morphology panel, *top images*). A through-plane phase-contrast acquisition shows the central MR jet (morphology panel, *right-hand middle image*). LGE imaging reveals extensive ischemic myocardial scaring (morphology panel, *right-hand bottom image*). The MR volume (MRvol) is quantified using the standard method: LV stroke volume (LVSV) minus aortic phase-contrast forward volume (AoPC). LVEDV, left ventricular end-diastolic volume; LVESV, left ventricular end-systolic volume; MRRF, mitral regurgitation fraction. (*From* Garg P, Swift AJ, Zhong L, et al. Assessment of mitral valve regurgitation by cardiovascular magnetic resonance imaging. Nat Rev Cardiol. 2020;17(5):298-312; with permission.)

and volumes by SSFP technique of CMR can be an integral part of a comprehensive assessment as a reference method and are needed for the decision making of a treatment plan (timing of surgery). Ventricular volumes are determined from a short-axis stack of 6-mm-thick to 8-mm-thick slices. They can be analyzed with off-line software, allowing endocardial and epicardial border tracing of both ventricles automatically or manually. Likewise, the Simpson method can be used to calculate ventricular volumes, ejection fractions, and myocardial mass.[36]

Flow Visualization and Quantification

Phase-contrast velocity encoding is a technique that uses velocity-encoding (VENC) gradients to generate a phase shift in the MRI signal, which is proportional to the velocity of the moving protons.[36] Four-dimensional-flow CMR allows for visualization of 2D velocity vectors in a designated plane, enabling a comprehensive assessment of the blood flow dynamics in the LA. Velocity vector visualization of LA flow coupled with cine CMR can help to understand the cause of the MR, similar to Doppler imaging acquired from echocardiography.[36] The MR jet cane be visualized using both cine and 2D phase-

contrast CMR. Quantification of mitral regurgitant volume and fraction is the recommended technique, and the MR volume can be calculated by 4 different methods: (1) Standard method and widely used: the difference between the LV stroke volume calculated using planimetry of cine SSFP images and the aortic forward volume obtained by phase-contrast images (Fig. 10); (2) the difference between the LV and RV stroke volumes calculated using planimetry of cine SSFP images; (3) the difference between the mitral inflow stroke volume and the aortic forward volume; and (4) direct quantification of MR flow by 4D-flow CMR with retrospective MV tracking.[35]

For the evaluation of patients with MR, late gadolinium enhancement (LGE) imaging to test viability should be performed in accordance with published guidelines.[37] Contiguous, short-axis, LV stack LGE imaging is needed, in addition to LGE in the 3 standard long-axis planes.

SUMMARY

The MV complex's proper function needs the integrity of leaflets, annulus, chordae, PMs, ventricle, and atrium. Functional, structural, or geometric distortion of 1 or more of these parts may cause valvular dysfunction. Therefore, a comprehensive evaluation with multimodality imaging is crucial. Echocardiography is the primary imaging modality for assessing the MV. Although roles of CT and CMR are increasing, echocardiography will serve as the first-line imaging modality for the diagnosis and serial follow-up in most cases. Cardiac CT scan acquires the images with the injection of contrast agents. Cine reconstruction methods using volume-rendered images are useful for visualizing the MV structure, including prolapse segments, vegetation, and dehiscence of the prosthetic valve. CMR provides a comprehensive evaluation of cardiac anatomy, function, and myocardial tissue characterization, and the usefulness to assess valvular heart disease, especially regurgitation. The utility of CMR evaluating valvular regurgitation has recently been adopted as part of the guideline. Finally, improved accuracy in the noninvasive assessment of MV and its related structures with multimodality imaging will ultimately translate to better management to improve outcomes for patients with MV disease.

CLINICS CARE POINTS

- Echocardiography is the primary imaging modality for visualizing the mitral valve. 3D imaging provides incremental value in assessing the severity of valvular heart disease and establishing its mechanism and is crucial for the guidance of percutaneous interventions.

- Roles of computed tomography and magnetic resonance imaging (CMR) are increasing. For the assessment of mitral regurgitation severity, CMR has recently been adopted as part of the guideline and become an established noninvasive imaging modality.

DISCLOSURE

The author has nothing to disclose.

REFERENCES

1. Nkomo VT, Gardin JM, Skelton TN, et al. Burden of valvular heart diseases: a population-based study. Lancet 2006;368(9540):1005–11.
2. Tumenas A, Tamkeviciute L, Arzanauskiene R, et al. Multimodality Imaging of the Mitral Valve: Morphology, Function, and Disease. Current Problems in Diagnostic Radiology. 2020. https://doi.org/10.1067/j.cpradiol.2020.09.013.
3. Berdajs D, Zund G, Camenisch C, et al. Annulus fibrosus of the mitral valve: reality or myth. J Card Surg 2007;22(5):406–9.
4. Kim DH, Heo R, Handschumacher MD, et al. Mitral valve adaptation to isolated annular dilation: insights into the mechanism of atrial functional mitral regurgitation. JACC Cardiovasc Imaging 2019;12(4):665–77.
5. Barlow JB. Perspectives on the mitral valve. Philadelphia: F.A. Davis; 1987.
6. Morris MF, Maleszewski JJ, Suri RM, et al. CT and MR imaging of the mitral valve: radiologic-pathologic correlation. Radiographics 2010;30(6):1603–20.
7. Ranganathan N, Lam JH, Wigle ED, et al. Morphology of the human mitral valve. II. The value leaflets. Circulation 1970;41(3):459–67.
8. Ho SY. Anatomy of the mitral valve. Heart 2002;88(Suppl 4):iv5–10.
9. Lam JH, Ranganathan N, Wigle ED, et al. Morphology of the human mitral valve. I. Chordae tendineae: a new classification. Circulation 1970;41(3):449–58.
10. Bax JJ, Debonnaire P, Lancellotti P, et al. Transcatheter interventions for mitral regurgitation: multimodality imaging for patient selection and procedural guidance. JACC Cardiovasc Imaging 2019;12(10):2029–48.
11. Zoghbi WA, Adams D, Bonow RO, et al. Recommendations for noninvasive evaluation of native valvular regurgitation: a report from the American Society of Echocardiography developed in collaboration with the Society for Cardiovascular Magnetic Resonance. J Am Soc Echocardiogr 2017;30(4):303–71.
12. Tsang W, Lang RM. Three-dimensional echocardiography is essential for intraoperative assessment of mitral regurgitation. Circulation 2013;128(6):643–52 [discussion: 652].
13. Lang RM, Badano LP, Tsang W, et al. EAE/ASE recommendations for image acquisition and display using three-dimensional echocardiography. Eur Heart J Cardiovasc Imaging 2012;13(1):1–46.
14. La Canna G, Arendar I, Maisano F, et al. Real-time three-dimensional transesophageal echocardiography for assessment of mitral valve functional anatomy in patients with prolapse-related regurgitation. Am J Cardiol 2011;107(9):1365–74.
15. Klues HG, Proschan MA, Dollar AL, et al. Echocardiographic assessment of mitral valve size in obstructive hypertrophic cardiomyopathy. Anatomic validation from mitral valve specimen. Circulation 1993;88(2):548–55.
16. Kim DH, Handschumacher MD, Levine RA, et al. In vivo measurement of mitral leaflet surface area

and subvalvular geometry in patients with asymmetrical septal hypertrophy: insights into the mechanism of outflow tract obstruction. Circulation 2010; 122(13):1298–307.

17. Chaput M, Handschumacher MD, Tournoux F, et al. Mitral leaflet adaptation to ventricular remodeling: occurrence and adequacy in patients with functional mitral regurgitation. Circulation 2008;118(8): 845–52.

18. Dal-Bianco JP, Aikawa E, Bischoff J, et al. Active adaptation of the tethered mitral valve: insights into a compensatory mechanism for functional mitral regurgitation. Circulation 2009;120(4):334–42.

19. Cobey FC, Swaminathan M, Phillips-Bute B, et al. Quantitative assessment of mitral valve coaptation using three-dimensional transesophageal echocardiography. Ann Thorac Surg 2014;97(6):1998–2004.

20. Machino-Ohtsuka T, Seo Y, Ishizu T, et al. Novel mechanistic insights into atrial functional mitral regurgitation-3-dimensional echocardiographic study. Circ J 2016;80(10):2240–8.

21. Carpentier AF, Lessana A, Relland JY, et al. The "physio-ring": an advanced concept in mitral valve annuloplasty. Ann Thorac Surg 1995;60(5):1177–85 [discussion: 1185–6].

22. Lee AP, Hsiung MC, Salgo IS, et al. Quantitative analysis of mitral valve morphology in mitral valve prolapse with real-time 3-dimensional echocardiography: importance of annular saddle shape in the pathogenesis of mitral regurgitation. Circulation 2013;127(7):832–41.

23. Song JM, Jung YJ, Jung YJ, et al. Three-dimensional remodeling of mitral valve in patients with significant regurgitation secondary to rheumatic versus prolapse etiology. Am J Cardiol 2013; 111(11):1631–7.

24. Blanke P, Naoum C, Webb J, et al. Multimodality imaging in the context of transcatheter mitral valve replacement: establishing consensus among modalities and disciplines. JACC Cardiovasc Imaging 2015;8(10):1191–208.

25. Koo HJ, Yang DH, Oh SY, et al. Demonstration of mitral valve prolapse with CT for planning of mitral valve repair. Radiographics 2014;34(6):1537–52.

26. Koo HJ, Kang JW, Oh SY, et al. Cardiac computed tomography for the localization of mitral valve prolapse: scallop-by-scallop comparisons with echocardiography and intraoperative findings. Eur Heart J Cardiovasc Imaging 2019;20(5):550–7.

27. Ionescu A, Fraser AG, Butchart EG. Prevalence and clinical significance of incidental paraprosthetic valvar regurgitation: a prospective study using transoesophageal echocardiography. Heart 2003; 89(11):1316–21.

28. Ruiz CE, Jelnin V, Kronzon I, et al. Clinical outcomes in patients undergoing percutaneous closure of periprosthetic paravalvular leaks. J Am Coll Cardiol 2011;58(21):2210–7.

29. Koo HJ, Lee JY, Kim GH, et al. Paravalvular leakage in patients with prosthetic heart valves: cardiac computed tomography findings and clinical features. Eur Heart J Cardiovasc Imaging 2018;19(12):1419–27.

30. Habets J, Tanis W, Reitsma JB, et al. Are novel noninvasive imaging techniques needed in patients with suspected prosthetic heart valve endocarditis? A systematic review and meta-analysis. Eur Radiol 2015;25(7):2125–33.

31. Kim IC, Chang S, Hong GR, et al. Comparison of cardiac computed tomography with transesophageal echocardiography for identifying vegetation and intracardiac complications in patients with infective endocarditis in the era of 3-dimensional images. Circ Cardiovasc Imaging 2018;11(3): e006986.

32. Koo HJ, Yang DH, Kang JW, et al. Demonstration of infective endocarditis by cardiac CT and transoesophageal echocardiography: comparison with intra-operative findings. Eur Heart J Cardiovasc Imaging 2018;19(2):199–207.

33. Beaudoin J, Thai WE, Wai B, et al. Assessment of mitral valve adaptation with gated cardiac computed tomography: validation with three-dimensional echocardiography and mechanistic insight to functional mitral regurgitation. Circ Cardiovasc Imaging 2013;6(5):784–9.

34. Song Y, Yang DH, Hartaigh BÓ, et al. Geometric predictors of left ventricular outflow tract obstruction in patients with hypertrophic cardiomyopathy: a 3D computed tomography analysis. Eur Heart J Cardiovasc Imaging 2018;19(10):1149–56.

35. Garg P, Swift AJ, Zhong L, et al. Assessment of mitral valve regurgitation by cardiovascular magnetic resonance imaging. Nat Rev Cardiol 2020; 17(5):298–312.

36. Mathew RC, Loffler AI, Salerno M. Role of cardiac magnetic resonance imaging in valvular heart disease: diagnosis, assessment, and management. Curr Cardiol Rep 2018;20(11):119.

37. Kramer CM, Barkhausen J, Bucciarelli-Ducci C, et al. Standardized cardiovascular magnetic resonance imaging (CMR) protocols: 2020 update. J Cardiovasc Magn Reson 2020;22(1):17.

Periprocedural Echocardiographic Guidance of Transcatheter Mitral Valve Edge-to-Edge Repair Using the MitraClip

Jay Ramchand, MBBS, BMedSci*, Rhonda Miyasaka, MD

KEYWORDS

- Mitral regurgitation • Echocardiography • Heart failure

KEY POINTS

- Transcatheter mitral valve repair using edge-to-edge clip has been established as an alternative to open surgical repair in primary and secondary mitral valve diseases.
- Optimal periprocedural imaging using transesophageal echocardiography is critical to determine procedural candidacy and ensure safe and successful implantation.
- Multiplanar reconstruction can be used to display all key mitral views, including the long axis, bicommissural, short axis, and 3-dimensional en face views.
- The use of this technique with and without color Doppler allows determination of MR mechanism and origin with precision.
- For optimal periprocedural imaging guidance, we recommend a detailed echocardiographic approach using the 7 steps outlined in this review article.

INTRODUCTION

In individuals with significantly increased surgical risk, a reduction of mitral regurgitation (MR) severity can be accomplished percutaneously by approximation of the anterior and posterior mitral leaflets, with transcatheter edge-to-edge mitral valve (MV) repair. The procedure is a percutaneous adaptation to the surgically performed Alfieri stitch and results in a double orifice valve (∞). Although the initial application of MitraClip was limited to patients with predominantly central MR and degenerative disease, recent clinical trials in addition to improved technical experience and advancements in 3-dimensional (3D) echocardiography has allowed successful application to those with noncentral MR and secondary valve disease.[1]

Optimal periprocedural imaging using transesophageal echocardiography (TEE) is critical to determine procedural candidacy and ensure safe and successful implantation. In this review, we present a step by step overview of echocardiographic imaging for transcatheter MV edge-to-edge repair using the MitraClip device.

MITRAL VALVE ANATOMY

A comprehensive appreciation of MV anatomy and surrounding structures is important to facilitate optimal imaging guidance for transcatheter edge-to-edge MV repair. A detailed discussion of this is beyond the scope of this review and has been covered elsewhere.[2]

In brief, the MV complex comprises the mitral annulus, anterior and posterior leaflets, chordae

---

This article originally appeared in *Cardiology Clinics*, Volume 39 Issue 2, May 2021.

Department of Cardiovascular Medicine, Heart and Vascular Institute, Cleveland Clinic, 9500 Euclid Avenue, Cleveland, OH 44195, USA

* Corresponding author.

E-mail address: ramchaj@ccf.org

https://doi.org/10.1016/j.iccl.2023.09.006
2211-7458/24/© 2023 Elsevier Inc. All rights reserved.

tendinea, and papillary muscles (Fig. 1). The annulus marking the hinge line of the valvular leaflets is D shaped rather than circular.[3] The aortic valve is in fibrous continuity with the anterior leaflet of the MV. The annulus opposite the area of valvar fibrous continuity lacks a well-formed fibrous cord and tends to be weaker and hence more significantly affected in annular dilation.

OVERVIEW OF DEVICES AND PROCEDURE

The MitraClip device (Abbott Vascular, Menlo Park, CA) is a clip made of 2 polyester-covered arms roughly 8 mm long and 4 mm wide that functions to grasp both the anterior and posterior MV leaflets (Fig. 2). The clip is delivered by means of a 24F steerable catheter and triaxial delivery system via a femoral venous and transseptal approach to reach the systemic side and thus the MV.

The MitraClip NT_R and XT_R systems were introduced in 2018 and are an updated version of the previous versions of MitraClip (MitraClip and MitraClip NT). The XT_R device has 3 mm longer arms (with 2 extra rows of frictional elements), that expand the reach of the device by 5 mm compared with the MitraClip NT_R device. In general, the NT_R system is favored in patients with short, restricted leaflets (functional MR) or if there is concern for smaller MV area (MVA). The XT_R device, is favored with degenerative MR with longer leaflet lengths, larger, wider flail width, and gaps. Indications and contraindications have previously been discussed elsewhere.[2,4]

MitraClip implantation is performed under general anesthesia owing to the need for a controlled environment that allows real-time and often prolonged TEE guidance. In addition, controlled breath holds can then be performed to maximize stability during leaflet grasping, a sensitive step of the procedure. In brief, after gaining transfemoral venous access, transseptal puncture (TSP) is performed to allow the Mitra-Clip device to access the left atrium, where it is aligned with the mitral pathology, and then advanced into the left ventricle. The MitraClip system is then withdrawn toward the MV with the clip arms open and approximated to both the anterior and posterior leaflets. The grippers are then lowered to trap the leaflets between the grippers and the arms. Finally, the arms are then closed to oppose the anterior and posterior leaflets. If necessary, the device can be reopened for adjustment before device release and final deployment. Detailed echocardiographic evaluation is divided into 7 main steps which is covered step by step elsewhere in this article.

Procedural Guidance
Step 1: preprocedure evaluation
After the initiation of general anesthesia, TEE should be performed to complete a quick preprocedural checklist (Table 1). The first step is to confirm MR mechanism and origin to ensure there are no significant changes compared with prior imaging that would alter the plan for device placement. The pulmonary veins should be assessed to evaluate for flow reversal. Mitral stenosis should be assessed with the MVA and

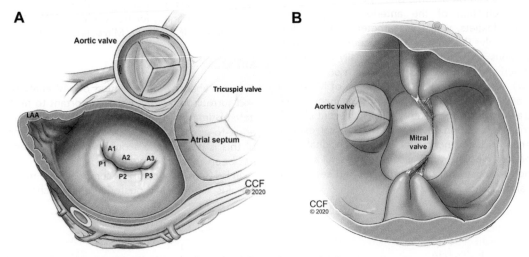

Fig. 1. MV anatomy. The MV as seen from the left atrial (*A*) and left ventricular (*B*) perspectives. The MV is composed of 2 leaflets, anterior and posterior, each of which is divided into 3 scallops, A1, A2, A3 and P1, P2, P3, as depicted. LAA, left atrial appendage. (Reprinted with permission, Cleveland Clinic Center for Medical Art & Photography ©2020. All Rights Reserved.)

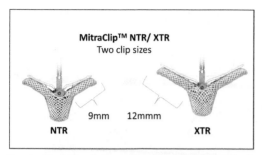

MitraClip™ NTR/ XTR
Two clip sizes

9mm   12mmm

NTR   **XTR**

Fig. 2. MitraClip devices. The MitraClip NT_R and XT_R systems introduced in 2018 comes in 2 sizes. The MitraClip XT_R device has 3 mm longer arms that expand the reach of the device by 5 mm over that of the MitraClip NT_R device. (MitraClip is a trademark of Abbott or its related companies. Reproduced with permission of Abbott, © 2023. All rights reserved.)

mean gradient. A MVA of less than $4.0\ cm^2$ is considered a relative contraindication to the procedure because deployment of the MitraClip may potentially result in significant stenosis.[4] Detailed indications and relative contraindications have been previously published and is beyond the scope of this review.[4] Preprocedure imaging should also establish baseline ventricular function, exclude intracardiac thrombus, and determine the presence of baseline pericardial effusion. The imager should also optimize and become familiar with key echocardiographic views to facilitate swift intraprocedural imaging. The key views include the bicaval, aortic valve short axis, bicommissural, long axis, and 3D views. An on-axis bicommissural view is crucial to understand the medial–lateral origin of the MR jet, and biplane imaging allows simultaneous visualization of a long axis view to understand

anterior and posterior leaflet anatomy and MR mechanism (Fig. 3A, B). A 3D en face view provides visualization of overall mitral anatomy, and pathology such as prolapse or flail (Fig. 3C). Multiplanar reconstruction (MPR) is a technique to simultaneously visualize multiple 2D imaging planes based on and along with a 3D dataset. The MPR planes can be aligned to display all key mitral views, including the long axis, bicommissural, short axis and 3D en face (Fig. 3D, E). The use of this technique with and without color Doppler allows a determination of the MR mechanism and origin with precision. A limitation to note when using 3D imaging is that there is some loss of spatial and temporal resolution compared with 2D imaging, and so 3D images should be used in conjunction with standard 2D views.

Step 2: transseptal puncture
The TSP is a critical step because the location establishes the trajectory of the device for the rest of the procedure. An optimal puncture will facilitate maneuvering of the device within the left atrium (LA) to establish an ideal alignment and trajectory with the MV (Fig. 4), whereas a suboptimal TSP can create multiple challenges that need to be overcome during the course of the procedure. The standard TEE views during TSP guidance are the bicaval view for visualization of the superior–inferior axis, the short axis aortic valve view for the anterior–posterior axis, and the 4-chamber view for measurement of TSP height (Fig. 5).

During the first step of the procedure, the catheter starts in the SVC. The interventionalist then slowly withdraws the catheter inferiorly into the right atrium to approach the interatrial septum (IAS). The primary imaging view at this point is the bicaval view to find the tip of the catheter, indicated by tenting of the IAS (see Fig. 5, arrows). The ideal TSP location is within the mid to superior portion of the fossa ovalis. Once the superior–inferior position is satisfactory, one moves to the short axis aortic valve view for anterior–posterior positioning. This maneuver can be done by changing the primary image to a short axis of the aortic valve or with the use of biplane imaging or live MPR (see Fig. 5). A posterior puncture is preferred to optimize height above the MV and the trajectory in the LA. Last, the height is measured, as visualized at 0°, in the mid esophageal 4-chamber view (see Fig. 5B). The ideal TSP height is 4 to 5 cm above the target grasping zone of the MV.

Note that very medial pathology requires a high TSP to allow enough room for the clip

Table 1
Immediate preprocedural checklist to be performed after anesthesia and endotracheal tube placement, before initiation of procedural steps

Immediate Preprocedural Checklist
1	Confirm MR severity, mechanism and origin. Become familiar with key TEE guidance views: bicommissural, long-axis, 3D en face, MPR, bicaval, AV short axis
2	Evaluate for pulmonary vein flow reversal
3	Measure MV gradient, and area using 3D planimetry
4	Rule out left atrial appendage thrombus
5	Evaluate for pericardial effusion
6	Evaluate interatrial septum for challenging anatomy

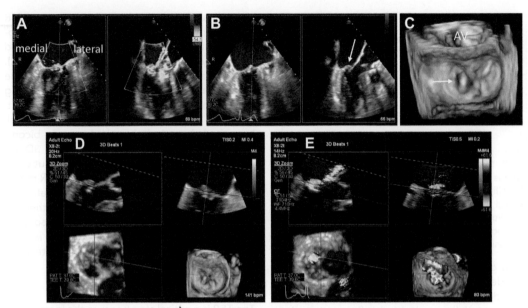

Fig. 3. Preprocedural evaluation of MR. (*A*) The MR origin is identified in the bicommissural view, which lays out the valve from medial to lateral. Biplane imaging is used to visualize the long axis view of the MR jet at this location. (*B*) Color Doppler is turned off to evaluate the underlying MV anatomy and determine the MR mechanism, in this case posterior leaflet prolapse and flail (*arrow*). (*C*) Three-dimensional en face view demonstrates P2 prolapse and flail (*arrow*). (*D*) Three-dimensional MPR shows all key views simultaneously, long axis (*upper left*), bicommissural (*upper right*), short axis (*lower left*) and 3D en face (*lower right*). (*E*) Three-dimensional MPR with color shows MR origin in all key views simultaneously (*E*).

delivery system (CDS) to bend back toward the septum without crossing into the left ventricle. Conversely, the lateral pathology is more forgiving with regard to TSP height (see Fig. 4B).

Once the proposed TSP site is satisfactory, the needle is advanced across the IAS. In addition to visualizing the needle on the left atrial aspect of the IAS, other supportive findings of successful puncture include resolution of tenting and/or visualization of bubbles in the LA.

It is important that the TSP needle is continuously monitored to avoid inadvertent damage to adjacent structures such as the LA free wall and aortic root.

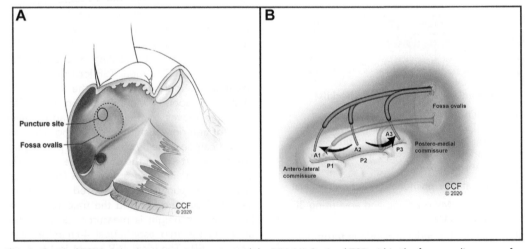

Fig. 4. Optimal TSP height showing trajectory toward the MV. (*A*) Optimal TSP within the fossa ovalis as seen from the right atrium. (*B*) Demonstration of TSP height for medial versus lateral pathology. If the TSP is too low (too close to the valve), there will not be room to adjust the device in the left atrium without crossing into the left ventricle. (Reprinted with permission, Cleveland Clinic Center for Medical Art & Photography ©2020. All Rights Reserved.)

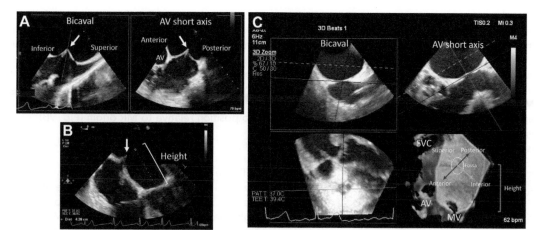

Fig. 5. Interatrial septal anatomy and guidance of the TSP. (*A*) The key views for guidance of the TSP include the bicaval view for superior–inferior axis (*left*) and the aortic valve short axis view for the anterior–posterior axis (*right*). The location of the needle is visualized by tenting of the septum (*arrows*). (*B*) The height is measured in the 4-chamber view from the tip of the mitral leaflets parallel to the septum until the level of the tenting. (*C*) Live MPR can be used to visualize all key views simultaneously. Movement along the superior–inferior and anterior–posterior axes in relationship to the MV height is demonstrated in the lower right image. Note that movement posteriorly, away from the AV, gains height above the MV. AV, aortic valve; SVC, superior vena cava.

Other anatomic challenges to consider include a patent foramen ovale, atrial septal defect or aneurysm, or septal hypertrophy.[5] Crossing through a patent foramen ovale risks tearing the IAS and also may create a trajectory of the guide hugging the anterior and superior wall of the LA. In the case of a septal aneurysm or mobile septum, applying pressure with the transseptal needle may bring it dangerously close to the LA free wall. In the presence of atrial septal hypertrophy, it is important to find the thin central portion of the fossa ovalis or use of a radiofrequency needle to facilitate puncture without exerting excessive force.[6]

After successful TSP, the guidewire is advanced into the left upper pulmonary vein or curled in the LA for stability. A 24F SGC with a dilator is then advanced to the septum (Fig. 6A).[4] It is important to monitor the tip of the guide crossing the septum, indicated by a double-density sign, as opposed to the dilator, which is cone shaped with multiple ridges This step can be performed with 2D imaging from the bicaval view or with live MPR (see Fig. 6A) When the guide has crossed the septum, the tenting disappears, and the double-density will be visualized clearly within the LA (Fig. 6B). It is important to lay out the length of the guide from the tip to the septum and at minimum the catheter should be advanced approximately 2 to 3 cm into the LA. This positioning should be monitored consistently throughout the procedure to prevent inadvertent retraction into the right atrium (Fig. 6C).

Step 3: advance the clip delivery system into the left atrium

The CDS is then advanced out of the guide until straddling (as seen on fluoroscopy), at which

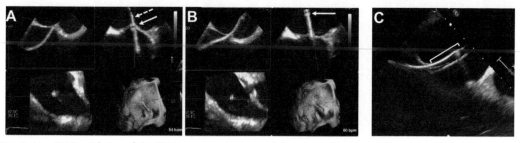

Fig. 6. Live MPR guidance of the SGC crossing the interatrial septum. (*A*) The guide tip is visualized on the right atrial side of the interatrial septum, indicated by the double density sign (*arrows*) along with tenting of the septum. The dilator is cone shaped with ridges (*dashed arrow*). (*B*) The guide tip has crossed into the LA with resolution of tenting. (*C*) The length of guide across the septum is measured.

point it can be steered down toward the MV. It is important to image the distal end of the CDS as it exits the SGC into the LA to avoid contact with the roof of the LA. Once the CDS is advanced sufficiently out of the guide, the clip is continuously tracked as it is steered down toward the MV. During this maneuver, the clip, LA appendage, and the warfarin ridge need to be visualized to ensure the clip does not catch the warfarin ridge or the left atrial appendage (Fig. 7A). Real-time 3D echocardiography can be useful to visualize the aforementioned structures in a single view (Fig. 7B).

Step 4: adjust the clip position and orientation

Once the CDS is advanced toward the MV, the next step is to position and orient the clip in the LA (Fig. 8). Manipulation within the left ventricle (LV) is minimized to prevent injury to the subvalvular apparatus. The key views for position the clip in the LA include the long axis view for anterior–posterior position (see Fig. 8A) and the bicommissural view for medial–lateral position (see Fig. 8B). Last, the clip orientation is visualized using a 3D en face view (see Fig. 8C) and is rotated clockwise or counterclockwise until it is perpendicular to leaflet coaptation. It is important to note that, if the clip is placed centrally, along A2 to P2, the clip orientation will be straight up and down; however, if the clip is placed medially, along A3 to P3, the clip typically requires counterclockwise rotation to remain perpendicular to the coaptation zone. Conversely, clockwise rotation is necessary when targeting lateral pathology, such as A1 to P1 (see Fig. 8C)

Biplane imaging allows simultaneously visualization of the long axis and bicommissural views.

Alternatively, live 3D MPR is a powerful tool because a single 3D dataset can be used to simultaneously visualize all key views, including the long axis, bicommissural, and short axis views, along with the 3D en face view (Fig. 9A). Before advancing into the ventricle, assessment using color Doppler should be used to confirm the clip position relative to MR origin (Fig. 9B).

Step 5: advancing the clip into the left ventricle and leaflet capture

With the clips arms and both mitral leaflets visualized, the clip is advanced across the MV into the LV. At this stage, it is critical to provide high-quality long axis images of the MV showing anterior and posteriorly leaflets as well as the anterior and posterior clip arms. This process can be done using single plane imaging, biplane imaging, or live MPR. Once in the LV, the clip is then slowly withdrawn back toward the LA until both leaflets are resting just above the clip arms in systole and diastole. The grippers are then lowered and one should pay close attention to the amount of anterior and posterior leaflets inserted in between the clip arms and grippers. The clip arms are then closed (Fig. 10). Historically, these steps are guided using single or biplane imaging. Recently, live MPR has shown to be a powerful tool to simultaneously monitor all aspects of clip position and orientation during this crucial stage of the procedure (Fig. 11).[7]

If, during the grasping sequence, it becomes difficult to image the clip, it is important to recognize that the clip position or orientation may have changed as it crossed the valve. The bicommissural view and 3D en face views may be helpful to evaluate for any changes in device location. When using live MPR, as opposed to

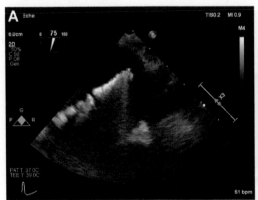
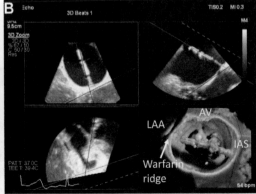

Fig. 7. Guiding the CDS within the LA. The clip must be continuously monitored to avoid injury to adjacent structures, specifically the roof of the LA, the warfarin ridge and the left atrial appendage. (A) 2D guidance keeping the tip of the clip in view to avoid injury to the LA free wall. (B) Live MPR guidance showing the CDS and key LA structures. AV, aortic valve; LAA, left atrial appendage.

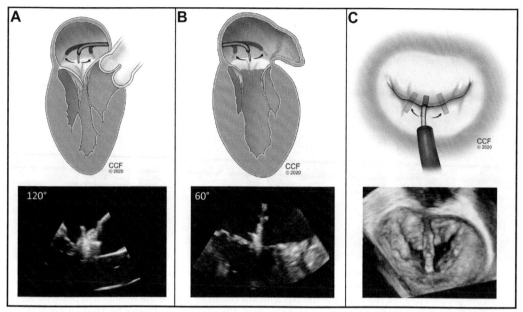

Fig. 8. Alignment of the CDS within the LA. (*A*) The long axis view is used for anterior-posterior adjustment, with anterior toward the AV and posterior away. (*B*) The bicommissural view is used for medial-lateral adjustment until the CDS is located above the target grasping zone. (*C*) The 3D *en face* view is used to adjust clip orientation with rotation of the clip clockwise or counterclockwise until perpendicular to leaflet coaptation. If the target is lateral, the clip typically needs clockwise rotation. Conversely, if the target is medial, the clip typically needs counterclockwise rotation. LA, left atrium. (Reprinted with permission, Cleveland Clinic Center for Medical Art & Photography ©2020. All Rights Reserved.)

single plane or biplane imaging, the clip position and orientation are monitored continuously, so that if changes occur, they are recognized immediately and corrected.

If leaflet capture is challenging, there are several maneuvers that can be helpful. If there is a large flail gap in systole, prolongation of

diastole with adenosine may be beneficial to bringing the leaflets closer together for grasping.[8] Conversely, if the problem is severe restriction of the leaflets in diastole, then rapid pacing to hold the leaflets closer together in the systolic phase may be helpful.[9] Breath-holding, with or without a Valsalva maneuver,

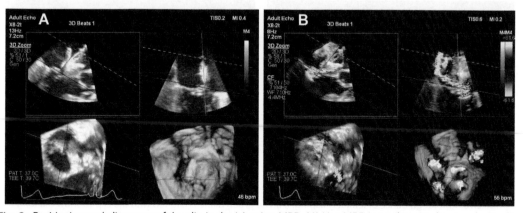

Fig. 9. Positioning and alignment of the clip in the LA using MPR. (*A*) Live MPR is used to simultaneously visualize all key views for alignment of the CDS in the LA: long axis view (*upper left*), bicommissural view (*upper right*), short axis view (*lower left*) and 3D *en face* lower right. The green plane is aligned with the clip arms in the short axis and 3D views to display the arms in the open position. (*B*) Once standard views are obtained and clip is aligned to target, color Doppler is added to confirm that the clip is aimed at the MR jet. LA, left atrium.

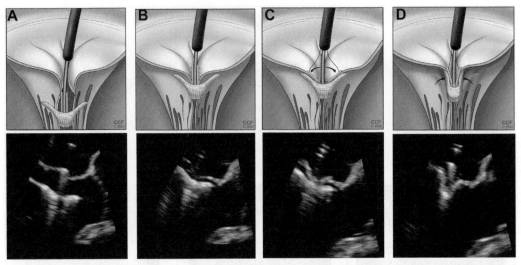

Fig. 10. Grasping sequence. (A) The clip is advanced into the LV. (B) The clip is slowly withdrawn back toward the LA until anterior and posterior leaflets are resting above clip arms. (C) The grippers are lowered to trap the leaflets between the grippers and the clip arms. (D) The clip arms are closed to appose the anterior and posterior leaflets. LA, left atrium; LV, left ventricle. (Reprinted with permission, Cleveland Clinic Center for Medical Art & Photography ©2020. All Rights Reserved.)

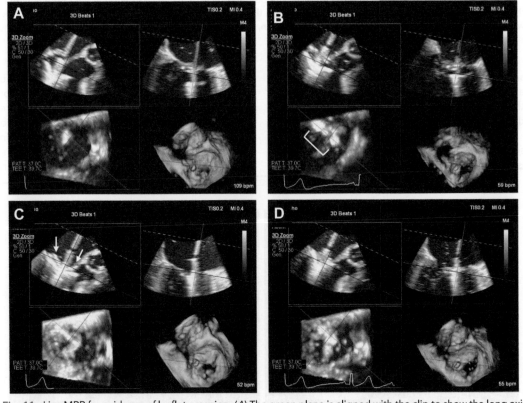

Fig. 11. Live MPR for guidance of leaflet grasping. (A) The green plane is aligned with the clip to show the long axis grasping view with clear visualization of both clip arms as well as anterior and posterior leaflets. (B) The clip is withdrawn back toward the LA until both mitral leaflets are resting on top of open clip arms. Note that within the blue plane, one can clearly visualize that the green grasping plane is aligned with the open clip arms (bracket) confirming on axis grasping views. (C) Grippers are lowered with leaflets inserted in between clip arms and grippers (arrows). (D) Clip is closed. Both anterior and posteriorly leaflets are immobilized.

may also be used to decrease the translational motion of the heart, which may in turn improve the ease of grasping.

Step 6: assessment of leaflet capture and residual mitral regurgitation

Once the leaflets are grasped, the next step is to determine if the device should be released (left in place) or repositioned. This decision is based on whether there is appropriate leaflet capture and adequate reduction in MR, while avoiding the development of mitral stenosis.

Leaflet grasp should be carefully assessed with multiple 2D and 3D views. The key 2D views are the long axis and 4-chamber views, demonstrating immobilization of both leaflets within the device (Fig. 12A, B). Another technique is to find the clip in the bicommissural view and then biplane through the device to show the long axis view in the orthogonal plane (Fig. 12C). Again, live MPR is a particularly useful too at this juncture, given its ability to

simultaneously display all the key views (Fig. 12D). Of note, a 3D en face view is helpful to show clip position and creation of a double orifice valve; however, this view alone cannot demonstrate degree of leaflet insertion. If the amount of leaflet insertion is questionable, one technique is to measure the baseline leaflet length before grasping and then compare it with the residual leaflet length outside of the clip after grasping (Fig. 13). Examples of poor leaflet capture are provided in Fig. 14. Single leaflet detachment can occur in between 1% and 5% of cases,[10,11] and so it is critical to confirm appropriate leaflet grasp before device deployment.

Residual MR is assessed using conventional methods,[12] including evaluation of proximal flow convergence and pulmonary venous flow pattern. A recent study has also demonstrated the utility of 3D vena contracta in assessing residual MR after MitraClip.[13] Invasive hemodynamics, including change in LA pressure after

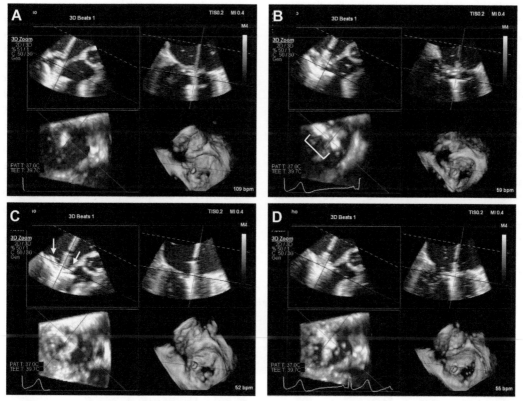

Fig. 12. Assessment of leaflet grasp. Grasp of anterior and posterior leaflets should be confirmed by demonstrating immobilization of leaflets within the device in multiple views, including (A) 0°, (B) long axis, (C) bicommissural view with biplane imaging, and (D) live MPR. Note that within the blue plane in panel B, one can clearly visualize that the green grasping plane is aligned with the open clip arms (bracket) confirming on axis grasping views. In panel C, capture and immobilization of the leaflets are demonstrated after lowering of the grippers (arrows).

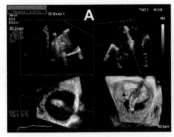
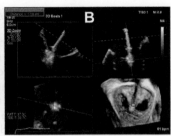
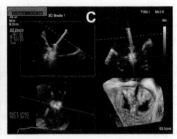

Fig. 13. Measurement of leaflet length to determine leaflet insertion. (*A*) The length of the posterior leaflet was measured before grasping, 1.5 cm. The remaining leaflet outside of the device was measured after grasping, 1.1 cm (*B*). The difference between leaflet length pre and post grasp was used to estimate the amount of leaflet inserted in the device. In this case, inadequate leaflet insertion was noted, only 4 mm. (*C*) Leaflet grasp was optimized and the posterior leaflet was remeasured, 0.8 cm, for over 0.6 cm leaflet insertion within the device.

MitraClip placement, is also an important metric to consider.[14]

Significant residual MR (>2+) should be evaluated carefully to determine the mechanism and etiology, as well as exact location, and specifically whether the origin is medial or lateral to the device. Either a bicommissural view with biplane imaging or live MPR are the best imaging tools to answer these questions (Fig. 15). A 3D view from the ventricle to visualize the proximal isovelocity surface area (MR origin) can be particularly useful in localizing residual MR.

If the residual MR is felt to be secondary to poor leaflet capture or incorrect placement, then the clip should be removed and repositioned. If clip position and leaflet capture are felt to be adequate, but additional pathology remains, then the anatomy should be evaluated to determine the suitability for additional clip placement. One must consider 2 factors in this situation: is the residual pathology graspable and is the residual MV orifice sufficient to accommodate an additional device without development of mitral stenosis. The target mitral gradient is less than 5 mm Hg because a mean mitral gradient of more than 5 mm Hg after the MitraClip is associated with adverse long-term outcomes.[15] If the gradient

is more than 5 mm Hg, one may try to slow the heart rate and reassess. In addition, 3D planimetry can be used to directly measure residual MVA. Because the 2 orifices may lie in different planes, each mitral orifice should be measured independently using 3D MPR, and then the 2 areas can be added for total residual MVA (Fig. 16). To answer the question of graspability of the residual pathology, one can simulate a potential grasping view by first localizing the residual MR with color Doppler, using either biplane imaging from the bicommissural view or live MPR, and then turning color off to understand the underlying leaflet anatomy (see Fig. 15). This assessment should be performed before releasing the clip. If an additional clip is not possible, then one may wish to consider adjusting the current clip for a better result.

In summary, clip placement is felt to be adequate for release if (1) good leaflet grasp at the target pathology (2) Mitral gradient and residual MVA is adequate (post clip MVA of >1.5 cm^2 with a mean transmitral gradient of <5 mm Hg), and (3) a significant decrease in MR by at least 1 grade to no more than moderate (2+) MR,[16] or if there is significant residual MR, an additional clip is anatomically feasible.

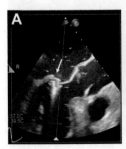
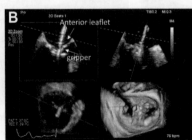
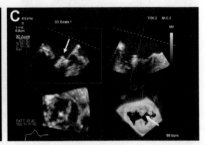

Fig. 14. Examples of poor leaflet insertion. Only tip of posterior leaflet captured (*A, arrow*). Anterior leaflet inserted above, not below gripper (*B*). Single leaflet detachment with clip only attached to anterior and not posterior leaflet (*C, arrows*).

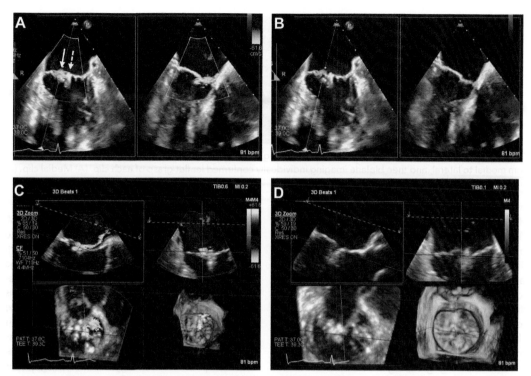

Fig. 15. Localization of residual MR and simulation of grasping view. (A) The bicommissural view demonstrates residual MR (arrow) medial to the device (dashed arrow). Biplane imaging shows the MR in long axis. (B) When color Doppler is turned off, MV anatomy can be assessed to understand mechanism of MR and suitability of anatomy for additional device. (C) Live MPR can be used to assess residual MR by aligning the green and red planes through the MR origin. (D) Color Doppler is then turned off to assess underlying leaflet anatomy at the MR origin to assess graspability at that location. Note that Live MPR shows a precise grasping view (green plane) compared with the biplane long axis view that appears off axis without clear LVOT and AV in view. AV, aortic valve; LVOT, left ventricular outflow tract.

Step 7: releasing the clip and closing views

After the clip is released, the MV should be reassessed because residual MR and the mitral gradient may change after tension from the CDS is removed. The LV ejection fraction may also decrease after clip deployment given the increased afterload as a result of decreased regurgitant flow into the LA. For this reason, with each clip, both before and after, the degree of residual MR, pulmonary venous Doppler and LV function should be reassessed.

Once satisfied with the mitral result, the CDS and SGC are withdrawn across the IAS under TEE guidance.

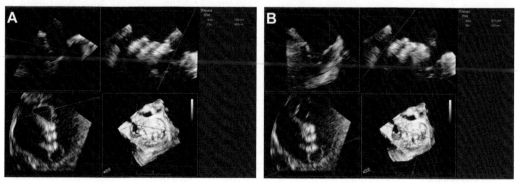

Fig. 16. Assessment of residual MVA by 3D planimetry. The (A) lateral and (B) medial orifices should be measured individually to calculate residual MVA.

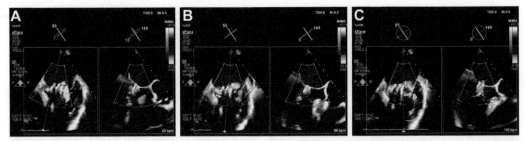

Fig. 17. Assessment of individual clips using biplane imaging. The bicommissural view was used to visualize 3 clips from medial to lateral, and then biplane imaging individually confirmed leaflet grasp of each clip. (A) Medial clip. (B) Middle clip. (C) Lateral clip.

SPECIAL CONSIDERATIONS

Placement of Additional Clips

Imaging guidance for placement of additional clips can be technically challenging because artifact from the first clip can make visualization of adjacent leaflets challenging. The additional clip is positioned and oriented in the LA, then advanced into the LV with arms closed (instead of open) to avoid disrupting the prior clip. It is important to ensure that the correct clip is being visualized during grasping and assessment of leaflet capture, because it is easy to confuse 2 adjacent clips, especially once closed. Both biplane (Fig. 17) and 3D MPR (Fig. 18) imaging are essential to allow detailed assessment of each individual clip. The sole use of single plane 2D imaging increases the possibility of evaluating the incorrect clip and missing inadequate leaflet capture.

Immediate Complications

The MitraClip procedure is overall a very safe procedure; however, there are several complications of which one must be aware. There is a risk of LA injury during TSP and with the movement of the equipment in the LA. For this reason, if hypotension occurs, one should quickly evaluate for the development of pericardial effusion and tamponade. When the clip is manipulated in the LV, it is possible for injury to the subvalvular apparatus to occur, which could lead to a chordal tear. This complication should be considered if MR changes in character or severity during the procedure. Another potential etiology of worsening MR is leaflet injury, such as leaflet tear, that can occur during grasping (Fig. 19). If MR worsens after clip release, then it is also important to consider the possibility of single leaflet detachment, which can occur secondary to either a leaflet tear or poor leaflet insertion (see Fig. 14C).

At the completion of the procedure, the residual iatrogenic atrial septal defect should be evaluated for size and direction of shunt flow. A previous study of a small series of patients showed an association of large residual defect (>10 mm) with increased morbidity and

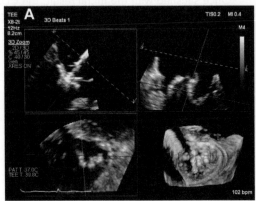
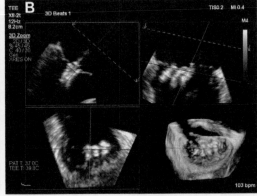

Fig. 18. Live MPR for placement of additional clips. (A) Live MPR was used for grasping during placement of a third MitraClip device laterally. The grasping plane (upper left) shows insertion of anterior and posterior leaflets within the arms and grippers. (B) Leaflet grasp was confirmed using Live MPR. All 3 devices are clearly seen on bicommissural (upper right) and short axis (lower left) views, with the long axis green plane (upper left) aligned to confirm grasp of anterior and posterior leaflets.

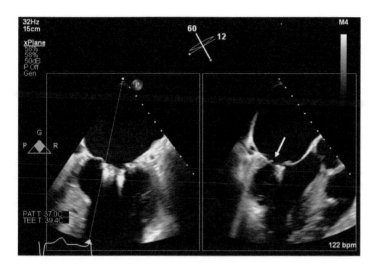

Fig. 19. Leaflet tear. Biplane imaging through the medial clip shows the grasp of this clip, which in this case demonstrates a leaflet tear (*arrow*), as indicated by the very short residual posterior leaflet with flail.

mortality, so atrial septal defect closure may be considered in these patients.[17] Significant right-to-left shunting with hypoxia is another indication for closure.

DISCLOSURE

The authors have nothing to disclose.

REFERENCES

1. Stone GW, Lindenfeld J, Abraham WT, et al. Transcatheter mitral-valve repair in patients with heart failure. N Engl J Med 2018;379:2307–18.
2. Ramchand J, Harb SC, Krishnaswamy A, et al. Echocardiographic guidance of transcatheter mitral valve edge-to-edge repair. Struct Heart 2020;4: 397–412.
3. Ho SY. Anatomy of the mitral valve. Heart 2002; 88(Suppl 4):iv5–10.
4. Wunderlich NC, Siegel RJ. Peri-interventional echo assessment for the MitraClip procedure. Eur Heart J Cardiovasc Imaging 2013;14:935–49.
5. Ramchand J, Harb SC, Miyasaka R, et al. Imaging for percutaneous left atrial appendage closure: a contemporary review. Struct Heart 2019;3: 364–82.
6. Tokuda M, Yamashita S, Matsuo S, et al. Radiofrequency needle for transseptal puncture is associated with lower incidence of thromboembolism during catheter ablation of atrial fibrillation: propensity score-matched analysis. Heart Vessels 2018;33:1238–44.
7. Harb SC, Krishnaswamy A, Kapadia SR, et al. The added value of 3D real-time multiplanar reconstruction for intraprocedural guidance of challenging MitraClip cases. JACC Cardiovasc Imaging 2020;13:1809–14.

8. Borgia F, Di Mario C, Franzen O. Adenosine-induced asystole to facilitate MitraClip placement in a patient with adverse mitral valve morphology. Heart 2011;97:864.
9. Hahn RT. Transcathether valve replacement and valve repair: review of procedures and intraprocedural echocardiographic imaging. Circ Res 2016; 119:341–56.
10. Maisano F, Franzen O, Baldus S, et al. Percutaneous mitral valve interventions in the real world: early and 1-year results from the ACCESS-EU, a prospective, multicenter, nonrandomized post-approval study of the MitraClip therapy in Europe. J Am Coll Cardiol 2013;62:1052–61.
11. Sorajja P, Mack M, Vemulapalli S, et al. Initial experience with commercial transcatheter mitral valve repair in the United States. J Am Coll Cardiol 2016;67:1129–40.
12. Zoghbi WA, Adams D, Bonow RO, et al. Recommendations for noninvasive evaluation of native valvular regurgitation: a report from the American Society of Echocardiography Developed in Collaboration with the Society for Cardiovascular Magnetic Resonance. J Am Soc Echocardiogr 2017;30: 303–71.
13. Avenatti E, Mackensen GB, El-Tallawi KC, et al. Diagnostic Value of 3-dimensional vena contracta area for the quantification of residual mitral regurgitation after MitraClip procedure. JACC Cardiovasc Interv 2019;12:582–91.
14. Siegel RJ, Biner S, Rafique AM, et al. The acute hemodynamic effects of MitraClip therapy. J Am Coll Cardiol 2011;57:1658–65.
15. Neuss M, Schau T, Isotani A, et al. Elevated Mitral Valve Pressure Gradient after MitraClip implantation deteriorates long-term outcome in patients with severe mitral regurgitation and

severe heart failure. JACC Cardiovasc Interv 2017;10:931–9.

16. Stone GW, Adams DH, Abraham WT, et al. Clinical trial design principles and endpoint definitions for transcatheter mitral valve repair and replacement: part 2: endpoint definitions: a consensus document from the mitral valve academic research consortium. J Am Coll Cardiol 2015;66:308–21.

17. Schueler R, Ozturk C, Wedekind JA, et al. Persistence of iatrogenic atrial septal defect after interventional mitral valve repair with the MitraClip system: a note of caution. JACC Cardiovasc Interv 2015;8:450–9.

Printed and bound by CPI Group (UK) Ltd, Croydon, CR0 4YY

03/10/2024

01040363-0013